Eating
Smartly

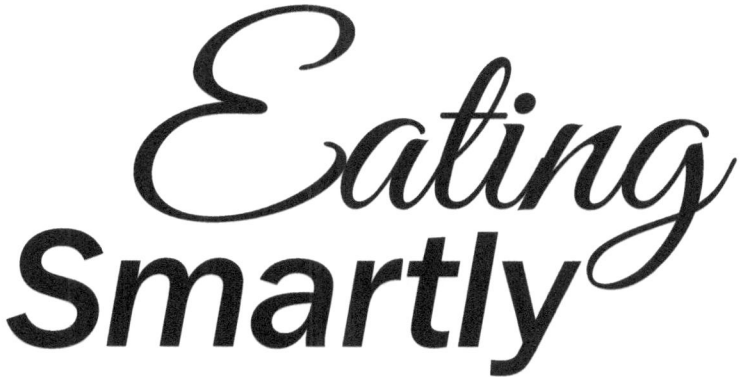

Eating Smartly

A Guide to Pursuing a Healthier Life
through Diet and Exercise

MIA NASSINI

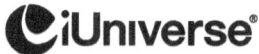

EATING SMARTLY
A Guide to Pursuing a Healthier Life through Diet and Exercise

iUniverse books may be ordered through booksellers or by contacting:

iUniverse
1663 Liberty Drive
Bloomington, IN 47403
www.iuniverse.com
1-800-Authors (1-800-288-4677)

ISBN: 978-1-5320-0259-5 (sc)
ISBN: 978-1-5320-0260-1 (hc)
ISBN: 978-1-5320-0261-8 (e)

Library of Congress Control Number: 2016912073

Print information available on the last page.

iUniverse rev. date: 12/15/2016

I dedicate this book to my Mom and Dad for their love and support and to my dearest, most powerful life coach, Tom, for his encouragements. To the future generation, I pray that you have plentiful, healthy food to eat with no side effects. There are thousands of food activists such as myself willing to fight to bring you the best of the best on your plate, and to your local communities.

Contents

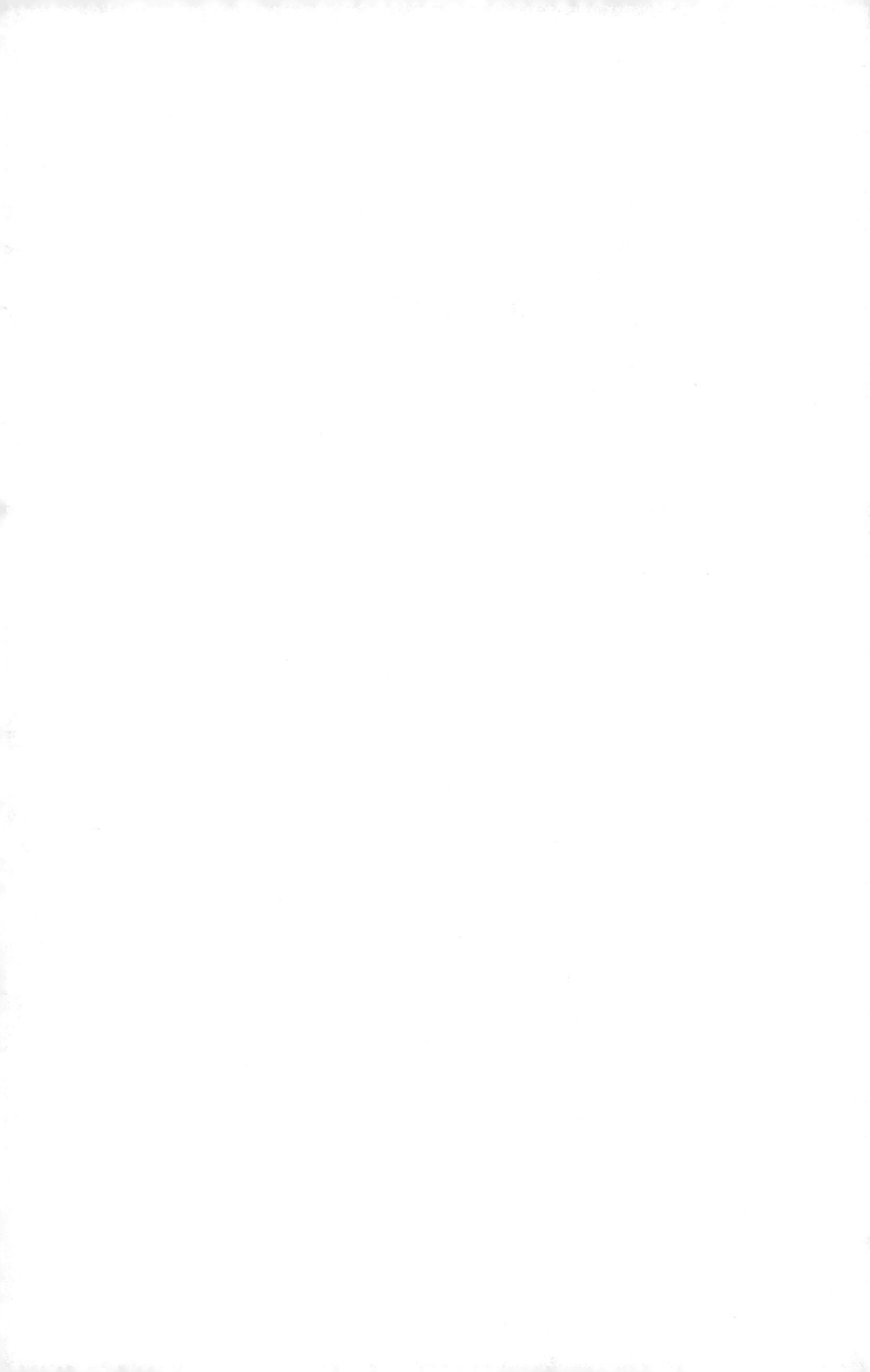

My Story

I came to United States a few years ago to further my education. Living by myself with no family to hang on to, I decided to indulge in free eating. Sometimes, being a student means living on a very tight budget. With the high cost of living in America and my lack of time, I barely had enough left for my groceries or for a home-cooked meal. I embraced the usual "American diet", meaning donuts in the morning, a box of pizza at lunch with a bottle of diet soda and Chinese takeout at night.

I lived that way for more than four years until I began to suffer severe headaches and constant blackouts. A friend of mine suggested I pursue the causes of the pain. With no health insurance, I was immediately rejected by a local hospital, but my friend called in a favor from a colleague of hers for a free MRI to determine the causes of my headaches. This was illegal, but my headaches were getting worst from day to night. My parents lived abroad and I was all by myself with no means and physical support from them.

The MRI revealed a brain tumor. Right upon hearing the news, I was devastated and shut myself away from my family, friends, and the rest of the world. It was the most difficult period. I was told that without treatment, I only had two years to live and that same sentence kept on ringing in my ears repeatedly. I quit my part-time job, spent most of my time at home and in school whenever I could. No health insurance would take a chance because I was what they considered a "lost cause". I started eating more and more of the comfort food and told myself that if I were to die from this illness, I should be by myself and not involve my family in my mistakes. Although they tried so many times to get in touch with me, I decided to stick to my dark place and kept on living in my misery. I passed out and threw up too many times to count.

The only meal I could keep down was the burgers and ice tea from my local fast food restaurants. Before I knew it, I went from a size 2 to size 18 in just eight months. I could barely fit into my usual outfits as life became worst for me. With my limited funds, purchasing new outfits was impossible. I wore the same pair of jeans and a couple of shirts that still fit to school and every other place for five months.

One day, I realized that I did not want to live this way; I wanted to live, I wanted to fight, I wanted to regain my health. I went to a bookstore and purchased every useful health and fitness book including DVD I could find and started following their instructions. Some of the books were useful, but others were just moneymakers-they would work for two weeks, then I would end up regaining my original weight, plus more on top of it!

Feeling down, but not out, I decided to do my own research. I became curious about where my meat and ingredients came from. I was also curious to know whether the cancer and the pain I was going through originated with what I was putting in my body. I started watching a lot of food documentaries and at the same time doing my own research to find the root of my disease and how to heal it safely and efficiently without causing any further harm to my body.

I was astonished with the information I discovered. After having discovered the roots and causes of my illness, I decided to change my ways and get my body healthy by consuming locally and organically grown foods. I decided to relive the days I have spent with my mother, a marvelous cook who up to now still uses only the freshest ingredients in her dishes.

It was not an easy process. I had the worst days of my life during the process, but eventually contacted my family and asked them for help. They stepped in quickly with some written recipes and portions that my mother recommended. With the help of my family, I was able to afford health insurance, but decided to wait five months and heal my body the natural way instead of opting for a chemotherapy or radiation. I told myself that whenever the outside of my body suffers an injury, it heals itself, so why couldn't the inside of my body do the same thing?

I purchased a juicer and everything else I needed to consume my food organically and healthily. I stopped consuming meat during that time and only lived on salads and vegetables juices. Five months later, I went ahead and signed up for a health insurance without mentioning any discovery of a tumor or any other pains for that matter.

The only thing my doctors were aware of was my headaches. They requested an MRI and in December of 2013, the most miraculous thing happened. The test came back clean; there was no sign of the brain tumor that I have previously been told would be the death of me. I was breathless, astonished and called it "My Christmas Miracle". Along with the miraculous disappearance of my tumor, I also shed a few pounds. My energy level was up, but the headaches continued, to the point where sleep became a treasure every night.

The pain was at times unbearable that I was hospitalized several times and had numerous medications, which I had to take to resume my daily routines. I became hopeless, threw away my pills and decided to only juice for two months, just with vegetables with an occasional apple add-on, jog every morning and consume at least 10 bottles of water daily. After my first week, my headache count dropped from 11 down to 4. I was able to resume my daily routines effortlessly and had more energy throughout the day. From there, I added more recipes to my diet, mostly French recipes and more juices that my mother recommended. I started reading labels before purchasing anything outside of my home. I prepared my meals every Sunday and stuck them in my fridge to discourage myself from embracing my old habits.

By June of 2014, I had dropped from 180 pounds to 135 pounds. I reduced my trips to the doctor's office and finally purchased the new outfits that I wanted. I went forward to starting my own company while finishing my doctorate from UCLA. I am currently juicing four times a year, but always stock my refrigerator with healthy foods. Instead of as a meal, I consume meat as a treat once a week usually on Saturdays. I lost weight naturally but have no regrets going through these experiences because it made me who I am today and I believe we are all build on our past experiences and mistakes. I made a vow to myself to always consider my body as an irreplaceable engine, which is why fueling it with proper food and care is the best way to live. I kept a dairy of my painful experiences then eventually became the book you are now reading. I hope you enjoy it and never go through my misfortunes. I am neither a nutritionist nor a physician to advise anyone to embrace my path, but all I can recommend is a proper care of your body. You only have one life to live; how you choose to live it is up to you!

Why Will *Eating Smartly* Work for You?

Eliminating unhealthy foods could push you to stray from your path; therefore, making your food choices healthy ones is the best way to get on track. This book lists fruits and vegetables that are high in fiber, which can contribute to blocking your hunger for long hours without resorting to unhealthy foods. Lean proteins are also listed to help boost your metabolism in various ways.

Furthermore, this book instructs you on how to pack your food to take to work or school in order to avoid the temptation of junk food from the vending machines. You also learn about how to package your foods for storage and add variations in your diet without hurting your weekly goals. With the massive amount of instructions and recipes, you will be less likely to get bored eating healthy!

Most importantly, *Eating Smartly* works well because it is realistic. Everything incorporated from breakfast to lunch is made affordable regardless of your financial status. This book contains a bonus list of organically grown farmers' market locations for healthy yet affordable groceries.

"*Eating Smartly* is written from real-life experiences and includes some ideas that you might not be aware of but that are very efficient. One of the secrets of great weight-loss success is the consumption of healthy foods without adding unnecessary carbohydrates and calories. This does not mean that consuming just broccoli or flaxseed every single day is the way to go; it means introducing delicious foods to your diet so that you do not miss your double cheeseburger from your favorite fast-food restaurant.

Section 1

The Mechanism of Eating the Right Foods

Many attempt to go through a diet without learning enough about what they are doing. This section teaches you about efficient methods and techniques to lose weight healthily, easily, and effortlessly. Its chapters are practical and easy to read! Furthermore, it exposes the macronutrients and micronutrients of some healthy ingredients to promote better health and weight loss for you and your family.

Before we begin, there is a series of questions that you would have to ask yourself. Answer these questions with a *yes* or *no*.

Four Questions to Ask Yourself:

1. Does my food come from a natural source?
2. Is my food high in micronutrients such as fiber, vitamins, minerals, and antioxidants?
3. Has this food lost its nutrients during processing?
4. Is this food high in sodium (salt), MSG, or any other items that could undermine my health (chemicals or trans-fats)?

Sample Motivation Chart.

In the chart below, state your motivations for losing weight and why shedding weight matters to you, including the number of pounds you would like to drop in your own chosen period of time.

To take this new habit to the next level and follow it weekly, I recommend purchasing a lined notebook for your future write-ups.

What is my motivation?
Why does weight loss matter to me and how many pounds would I like to shed?

Sample Daily Planner

In a daily planner, jot down everything you consumed during the course of a day, even if it is not in your diet. It will be a reference for your progress or regression. This will allow you to be your own judge, instead of being told what to do or what might be hurting your diet and weight loss.

Due to the limited space in this chart, I recommend purchasing a notebook for your future daily listings.

Breakfast	
Snack (optional)	
Lunch	
Snack (optional)	
Dinner	
Evening Snack (optional)	

Weight Loss and Its Mechanisms

Eating Smartly starts with different aspects of weight loss, with the incorporation of different strategies that can be used in one's daily routines. Each topic discussed differentiates from others by giving you most of the tips and tricks to get your weight under control and embrace a good healthy life. Section 1 of the book discusses the issues of stress, how to avoid overeating, the true nature of weight loss, various fruits and vegetables to consume, and many other nutrition-related aspects.

This book will walk you step-by-step through how to reduce your weight easily and healthily without hurting your body or health. There are also some breakfast, lunch, and dinner recipes included in some of the chapters to help you on your path to great health. This book will be helpful only if you persevere enough to get the success you desire. Do not forget to consult your physician before starting any new or unfamiliar weight-loss regimen.

Have You Ever Wished you could...

Drop a size or two in a matter of weeks?

Have almost all the tips you might need in one book to help you achieve success?

Stay motivated with your diet without feeling the urge to quit?

Have more energy from the foods you consume?

Have a weight-loss book that includes almost anything you need, from nutrition to physical exercises that actually work, along with illustrations?

Have fun while dropping sizes along with your family and friends?

Have admirers left to right noticing the "New You"?

Set goals and meet them more easily?

If you answered "yes" to some of these questions, it means that you are ready to learn more about how to get yourself healthy again. I hope the tips and tricks in this book will help you embrace your way to becoming the healthier person that you desire to be.

Introduction

Next time you're around a group of people, listen to their discussion, especially the women. You'll be amazed how often the conversation turns to either weight loss or dieting. Whether it is for a special occasion or to fit into that special outfit, we all turn to the latest fad for a quicker result. But does it help us accomplish what we seek? That is the question you have to ask yourself when watching a TV commercial touting the next "can't miss" diet. I call those fad diets "*The Illusion Effect*". We invite our friends and family to join us in "*The Illusion Effect*" and whenever it doesn't work, we get disappointed and move on to the next one. Each time you turn on your television, you see all those celebrities with slimmer bodies causing us to belittle ourselves! On the other side, there are the advertisements that promote cheap foods indulging Americans, especially those with lower wages, to purchase them in order to feed themselves and their families. Two out of three Americans are overweight or obese, and children comprised one-third of that figure. Per year, Americans spend more than $100 billion on fast food alone, and $60 billion a year on weight loss solutions. We are constantly bombarded by advertisements telling us that they can make you thin by using their various products in a shorter amount of time. There is this idea that weight can be lost magically without any major effort on our part.

The industrial food system is making us sick! Diabetes is on the rise and sadly, more individuals succumb to food-related diseases each year in this country. For most processed food manufacturers, the concept is to sell a huge amount of food at a low price. World War II caused two shifts in the social pattern. The first shift was due to soldiers who were weakened and dying by lack of food. A way had to be improvised in order to keep them healthy and alive. Americans have to figure out a possibility to transport food to the soldiers and the best way was to freeze and package it. Taste wasn't much of a concern at the time, the main goal was portability. Tons of foods were produced each day, and led to the idea of frozen foods in the US-making all manner of food available without spending as much money to produce a high quality product. The second shift was due to the lack time women had during WWII. Since most of the men were fighting, women worked outside the home. They were working overtime to support their families, therefore giving them little to no time to prepare a proper family meal. These two shifts gave birth to what we know today as "Food Industrialization". The portions of our foods are measured on transportability rather than health concerns. Monosodium glutamate (**MSG**), oil and sugar began making appearances in processed food, making those foods more appealing, in other word, addictive. Many people started consuming more and more of those foods, causing the processed food business to boom, and encouraging those companies to create more of what we now call "Killer Foods."

"Obesity, diabetes, heart disease, high blood pressure are all diet related health issues cost this country more than $120 billion each year," said US First Lady Michelle Obama. Weight gain is a lifestyle choice and can be eradicated by consuming the right foods. In 2009, more than 200,000 Americans made a life-changing or a lifesaving decision to reduce their weight with surgery. Based on current projections, by 2018, 40% of the population will be considered obese, and the cost of obesity related treatment will more than double its current price to $344 billion in health care costs alone. This could bankrupt the country There are a lot of obese children in the country and if not stopped, the next generation could also be seriously affected, making America an even unhealthier country. Most kids have been overweight their whole lives, and it is very difficult for them to let go of their old habits. Therefore, it is up to the parents to help make the change.

By teaching children how to eat healthy at a young age, they will be most likely to turn to better options instead of *"embracing the fast food lifestyle"*. You don't have to go to the best restaurants to get good food!

farmers markets are around the country to encourage the consumption of healthier foods regardless of your budget. I have listed some of them at the end of the book and I hope you will find them useful to feed your family instead of running to the nearest fast food restaurant around the corner. If we don't break up the chain and understand the decision that we make, we will keep on holding the trophy of an unhealthy nation. I am neither an expert nor a nutritionist, I am just a simple student who became sick due to my own bad diet and decided to write a journal, which then became the book you are now reading. I went through most of "*what works and what does not.*" I am not a "*know it all gal,*" but I have swallowed far too many pills and decided to put them behind and move forward. This book contains ingredients, recipes, and a fitness routine that worked for me. I hope you enjoy my findings and see better results in your overall health.

The book is split into three sections. The first section is about the importance of good nutrition (charts of various fruits, proteins and alcohol including their nutrient contents, portions and calories). The second section of the book contains healthy recipes to eliminate boredom in your food selection. The last section includes fitness tips and tricks with illustrations for a good workout regimen without a gym membership!

Let's have fun and live healthily!

Enjoy!

Chapter One

The Impact of Stress

For most people, obesity is a solution to being stuck in an unwanted situation. That is the reason why I attacked stress at the beginning of the book before we went on with the solutions to obesity and nutrition. A lot of us tend to turn to food whenever we are under stress. Food eases our hardships for a moment and fills a void. But, hardships cannot be resolved through food. Every time you experience an emotional stress, it activates chemistry pushing you to seek more and more of the food we commonly refer to *comfort food*. There are two neurochemicals responsible for obesity and unhealthy appetites: Cortisol and epinephrine. These two chemicals are there for our protection and their No. 1 reaction towards stress is fat storage. Cortisol is a product of adrenaline. The more stress you experience; the more cortisol you produce.

Cortisol in a sense communicates with the brain to *eat* and your belly to *store*. The *"eat and store"* phenomena increases whenever you are facing a marital, financial, or family issues. Being under stress means eating, and with the vast availability of fast food, it is easier and cheaper to indulge on food, which sadly does not solve our current challenges. Weight does not come from having a bad diet and cortisol alone; sleep deprivation and dehydration also can be the cause of your weight gain. Stress increases fluid retention, thus to avoid this unwanted phenomena, you need to identify the real causes of your stress and fix them before going ahead with your weight reduction. Life can be full of stress; it is up to us to make sure it is reduced to a minimum or eliminated. Some children tend to turn to food to overcome the circumstances they might be experiencing in school or at home in some cases. Parents, loved ones, even counselors in this case have to step in and help them overcome their worries. There are thousands of clinics willing to help children relieve their worries and get them healthy again. Exercising regularly also helps reduce stress and at the same time burns calories in the process. Physical exercise increases your good hormones and promotes a good mental clarity throughout your day. Taking a walk three to four times a week is as good as an anti-depressant medication. Anything that is pleasurable that isn't eating, smoking, drinking or taking drugs generally decreases your stress hormones.

Visualization is a way to push your subconscious and unconscious mind to accomplish your desires. Pictures are like a hidden language; they are really effective and promote an efficient method of healthy living. Hold up a picture of the body you want to be in front of your face for 30 seconds or more; then let your subconscious mind absorb it. Finally, close your eyes and see yourself in that body, walking or doing what you want, and your subconscious mind will follow suit. It is that simple! This small exercise helps you achieve results faster than intended. Most activities you will be performing will be unconsciously made, thereby leading to a great body figure.

Stop treating yourself badly whenever you are in a condition you despise. Treat yourself as you want others to treat you. Whenever you take care of yourself; you realize that you are precious, and that energy goes around everyone you meet, making your life not just livable but wonderful. When you love yourself, you will avoid putting on excess weight and take better care of your body. If you hold the sentence; "I am worthless and ugly," you will never do anything fruitful to make yourself happy. A life coach; Dr. Tom, once told me: "If God made you, you are beautiful and wherever you are in life, is purely based on the choices you make daily." There was a point in my life when I became helpless and the only comfort I had was my emotional eating. That was the comfort I could find in the world. I even tried on multiple times to take my own life. Life was not fun at that point. It wasn't until I woke up one day and said *enough* that I was able to take control of my life. Everything I had could no longer fit the body I was in. I had to purchase larger sizes. I went from a size zero to a size sixteen in less than a year. A couple of months later, my life coach reached out to me and helped *get on my feet*. You don't really have to have a life coach to help. All you need is your family or those around you who care! They are available to help *get you on your feet.*

That statement is so powerful that no matter what goes on in my life, I tend to take care of myself in a way that I want others to treat me. Everything starts with you loving yourself! Every day when I get up and see this statement, I instantly become fulfilled. Recite a good message every morning and night before going to bed. This is the greatest accomplishment you will ever make. Self-love is so powerful that it wires the healthy cells in your body, making you healthier than you have ever been. Stress can affect our lives negatively in many ways. If you have a lot of stress in your life, it can affect your relationships, your focus, your productivity, and even your health! That's why it's so important to learn to relieve and reduce stress in your life before getting on to your desires. Reducing or eliminating your stress before weight reduction is a stepping stone to obtaining a healthier self. Stress is the primary cause of any unhealthy eating; therefore, to see potential results and prevent a future weight gain, use the techniques provided below, and you will find it easier to reduce your stress, have the ability to stick to a healthy diet, and live a better life. Your body is designed to be healthy; grab it and move on!

Basic Tips to Relieve Stress in Your Environment

Managing stress in today's world can be a hard task to accomplish. Yet it is not hard if you are aware of what to do in the presence of a stressful situation. Stress negatively impacts your body and your mind. Knowing what causes your stress and how you can deal with it can greatly improve your health. An efficient system of personal organization can significantly lessen the stress you experience. Stress is usually the result of forgetting to carry out an important task or locate an unknown solution, which subsequently induces feelings of frustration and tension. The feeling of control over your own life will make your efforts at organization well worth the time invested. You must understand the situations that create your stress before you can handle them effectively. These are some basics steps and suggestions to lower your stress.

- An efficient system of personal organization can lessen the stress you experience. Organization is essential for managing anxiety-based stress. Most people tend to be disorganized, which causes confusion and frustration and which inevitably leads to anxiety and later stress. Simply being organized, whether at work or at home, can cut back on the anxiety and stress you experience. Work out all problems that you may experience through time management, especially when it comes to big projects. If you have a large project to do, break it down into small steps that you can handle. If you have everything laid out well, your stress level will greatly decrease compared to contemplating the project in full. When you keep yourself organized, you can lower your stress and complete the job effectively.

- The most important aspect in relieving stress is to reduce your caffeine intake! A large intake of caffeine can increase the levels of cortisol in the body. By decreasing your caffeine intake, you will naturally decrease your stress levels. Start maneuvering your way into drinking decaf coffee, and stay away from caffeinated sodas and other unhealthy beverages as well. Dropping caffeine all at once can cause headaches, so you might have to do this progressively or try drinking a cup of tea.

- To quickly relieve your stress, pay attention to your breathing! Make sure that you are breathing from your abdomen, not your chest. Take slow, deep breaths and make sure that your abdomen rises and falls accordingly. This will help get more oxygen into your blood, which will help reduce your level of stress. Everyone has different coping mechanisms, and you should develop them to reduce your stress levels. Consciously employ healthy coping mechanisms, like thinking positively about yourself whenever you sense difficulties. Positive thinking means a positive outlook, which enables you to have a different perspective compared to what stress might dictate.

- Most people experience stressful times in their lives, and some may cope with stress better than others. If you have a hard time dealing with your day-to-day stress, find five minutes a day to stop and clear your mind of your daily burdens. The efficient way to lessen your stress throughout your day is to meditate, especially in the morning before any other activity. This can be a great way to not only relax your body, but also clear your mind of everything that might be causing your stress. Consider buying audio tapes or books to assist you with different ways of meditation. Meditating and deep breathing in and out slowly through the mouth will work wonders to ease your stress levels, especially in the morning! Furthermore, many do not get the proper amount of vitamins into their daily diet. Taking a multivitamin can take care of this, and it is the best possible scenario for taking care of yourself and reducing stress in your daily life. If you take stress-control formulas, their content of vitamins is insufficient to lift your mood, and therefore these types of formulas should be avoided. Multivitamins are the key! Getting them from a natural source is a healthy habit. You can refer to my vegetable juicing recipes for a great morning boost!
- In case you continue to experience stress at work, listening to the music of your choice offers greater benefits. Be sure to play lower-key tones, as this will help soothe you. If a more upbeat music choice is made, it should be cheerful and happy. The right song can instantly lift your mood and help relieve stress. Keep a music player and headphones close by with some of your favorite songs at all times. When the stress becomes overwhelming, throw on your headphones and take a 10-15 minutes break and relieve your tension. Another action you can undertake is to imagine yourself at the beach, or any other tranquil environment. Visualizing is a great stress reducer in itself! The next time you begin to feel overwhelmed, take 5 minutes and imagine yourself in a soothing bath, on a sun-drenched beach, or in a beautiful forest. You may find the stress a little less overwhelming. Most importantly, search for sounds that can soothe your stressful day; get a table-top fountain. The sound of running water is therapeutic in calming the mind. These fountains come in all sizes and can be conveniently

placed on a table at home or in the office. So whenever you feel stress, just have some quiet time and listen to your mini-waterfall.

- To help you manage your stress, you should make time for relaxation and enjoyment. Do not carry all the worries of the world on yourself. Change the way you think and your attitude; let yourself relax. If you regularly make time for relaxation and enjoyment, you will be in a better position to handle the inevitable stress that will come your way. So take time to relax and you'll feel better, which will lessen the number of stressful situations you encounter. Replace unhealthy habits with healthy, productive ones. For example, if you tend to overeat when stressed, you should instead consider exercising. By replacing unhealthy coping strategies with healthy ones, your body will be able to stay strong and be better equipped to deal with daily stresses. Mix up a stress-reducing potion. Homeopathy can be a great way to reduce stress. Spearmint oil, for instance, can be a stress reduction method. Whenever you feel stressed out, dab a little on your temples and neck. You will be amazed how much relief you can find from simple remedies like this. Investigate it and see if it's right for you. Remedies that are all-natural and safe to use will have a good track record of effectiveness with many users.

- Another remedy is to fix your posture! People who are unhappy and stressed tend to have poor posture, which lessens the amount of oxygen going into their brain. This makes your thoughts more negative and also causes muscle aches. By standing up straight, you get more oxygen into your brain and you feel instantly better.

- Cultivating close relationships is a necessary part of life, but that doesn't mean it is always easy to do. Pets generally require less from you; consequently, they can be very relaxing. Interacting with a cherished pet can provide a rewarding break in your day, and the interaction also carries health benefits. Even if you don't have a pet, go to a friend's or neighbor's house and pet his or her animal for a few minutes; even just a few seconds of petting an animal will reduce your stress. Having a dog waiting for you at home with his or her tail wagging can be a great boost after a hard, stressful day at work. Even just having a fish can really improve your mood.

But don't take on a pet if you're not going to be able to care for it. Another way to cultivate relationships is to call an old friend to whom you have not spoken to for a long time and catch up. This will bring back the memories that you have had with him or her, which will make you feel great for the rest of the day. Additionally, when you are trying to cope with a large amount of stress, make sure that those close to you are aware that they are not the cause. Your friends and family, especially your spouse and children, can otherwise get the feeling that they have done something bad. You should own your stress. It is your condition, and you need to make sure that the people in your life whom you love and care about don't have to suffer along with you unnecessarily.

- Go online and check out different classes that are available in stress management. There you will be dealing with professionals who can help guide you with important tips to implement in your everyday routine. This will go a long way toward putting you in a better state of mind during the day. In case it does not give you the satisfaction that you require, a good tip that can help reduce your stress is to spend some time away from home for a week or two without a computer in hands. It can be very tempting to get on the Internet, but the objective of you getting away is to spend time by yourself. Most importantly, stop worrying about others and what they are or are not doing! You only have control over your own actions. Worrying about what other people are doing will constantly stress you at all time! Stop it and enjoy your life for a change!

- Examine how you deal with stress. Then you can think of ways to cope with it better. Track how you respond to stressful situations over a few weeks. Remember and evaluate your response to each stressful event and ask yourself if you handled it in an effective and healthy manner. If your responses were not as healthy as they should be, you can develop new ways of coping with your everyday stress. One aspect that usually leads to stressful behaviors is anger. Properly express your anger! It is a big part of stress management. When you get upset, you do not want to work yourself up and raise your blood pressure. Learn some safe techniques to deal with your anger and keep your stress level to a minimum. One simple way is to lay out your work clothes for the next day. It can give you a better start in the morning and provide you a few extra minutes to relax as well. Another way to relieve your anger is to talk about your problems once in a while with friends, but do not place yourself at the center of the relationship. Friends will always be there to listen, so it is vital to use this option to help relieve your stress and anxiety. But in any case, be wary of overburdening your friends with daily discussions of your life stressors and complex issues. An additional effective way to deal with stress is to keep a journal. Keeping a journal can go a long way in alleviating stress since it is an outlet for letting go of your stresses. Writing down your thoughts, for instance, in a formal journal or indulging in a "free writing" lets things out instead of bottling them up inside. This technique is a great way to relieve stress or anger.

- Develop an exercise regimen that will help minimize your stress hormones and neurochemicals. Exercise is an excellent first step in a program designed to relieve stress. Our bodies are programmed by centuries of evolution to flee in the face of stress. We can use this aspect of our evolution to our advantage; therefore, exercise at least three to five times each week for thirty minutes each session. The exercise can be anything from running to swimming to simply taking a daily walk. Physical activity has the benefit of releasing endorphins, chemicals that enhance your mood; making it a great way to de-stress at the end of a hectic day, and at the same time, get your heart rate pumping! Running is one of the absolute best activities you can do to help reduce stress. Not only does it help you to clear your mind, but it also releases endorphins into your body to help you feel more relaxed. It's not called a *runner's high* for nothing. Activities such as walking, tennis, running, swimming, or biking are really important, not only for weight loss but for your mind as well. Stress-related chemicals are burned off during exercise, and it is healthy for you, especially your heart! Even though running or other forms of exercising may seem like a really annoying experience, with time you may learn to love it. Try to keep an open mind about exercise, and you will see that it helps you feel less stressed, as well as much more energized throughout the day. If you are not the kind of person who enjoys running, then you can consider some type of martial art. The act of hitting an object or another person in an appropriate context can really help ease the desire to hit people in the absolute wrong situations in life.

- Stress is a double-edged sword that can cause extreme exhaustion while also causing the inability to fall asleep. To get a good night's sleep, take a nice warm bath immediately before bed. Relax your body in the water one bit at a time and let your cares drain away with the bathwater. Secondly, give your brain enough time to unwind before you go to bed. If your brain is still really active when you go to bed, you will find yourself worrying about everything you are supposed to do, which will leave you feeling stressed and unable to sleep.

As discussed, stress can have a negative effect on your mental and physical health. Hopefully, this advice given will not only help you identify the causes of your stress, but also help you sort it out your issues and help you live a happier and healthy life. Live your life according to the things you learn in this chapter, and you can diminish the amount of stress in your life as a whole. There are no reassurances when it comes to advice; ultimately it is up to you. You want to make sure that you remember all of the tips presented to you and be sure to look back at the chapter if you sense the need. There's no shame in rereading some of these tips if they are detrimental to your health. Now that you are armed with the knowledge of stress, it is time to introduce a good nutrition plan in your life. Keep reading!

Chapter Two

General Nutrition 101

"Let food be thy medicine." Hippocrates stated this sage advice more than 1,000 years ago. We have become creatures of convenience; we spend more on luxury cars or designer brands than our food. We were taught that food should be quick and ready within 15 minutes or less. Commercially based products are the ones that trigger the bad eating in this country. Unfortunately, beneath the appealing packaging, lurks foods that are high in fat, sucrose, and many other unhealthy components adding more to the obesity epidemic in America.

In the 1960s, the number of food franchises exploded in the United States as busier Americans started feeding themselves with those foods as a convenient way to get nourishment during brief breaks in their routines. With the introduction of fast foods, the rate of American cancer and other high cholesterol diseases began to rise. As a result, in 1971, President Richard Nixon introduced the "war on cancer campaign". Many medical procedures are on the road to discovery, including cures for breast cancer. Currently, there are more obesity related diseases compared to the time of our great grandparents. Individuals associate third-world countries with poor nutrition and poor health but the truth is that those countries grow and purchase their foods locally rather than importing them. Only a small fraction of their daily condiments are imported. This life choice improved their health with lower rates of obesity and cardiovascular diseases. We go to the supermarket and purchase all the vegetables we can find, not knowing that 50% of nutrients will be destroyed while cooking our food. If you consume at least 51% of your food raw, (most might find it undoable), we will become healthier than ever. Nutrition is not related to individual nutrients as we are taught on packages, but it comes as a whole to protect and defend the body from toxins or rather sicknesses. Healthy eating can help prevent cancer. Everything comes down to you! It is really important to take care of your body instead of spending your money on other things at the expense of your health. The best way to balance or adapt a healthy lifestyle is to consume more foods that are rich in healthy fat and high in fiber which can be potentially inexpensive due to the increasing numbers of farmers markets today!

The consumption of intact food is really essential to the nourishment of our cells, brain and many other parts of our body. When the body is not given what it needs, it weakens, and consequently it contracts more sicknesses, which means more money for the health industry. There are several key areas of nutrition that are really important for our body especially for a productive day. One of them is the consumption of vitamins. Vitamins are really significant to treat and heal our bodies; unfortunately, we do not consume enough of them, especially Vitamin C. Vitamin C is especially good for use as an anti-toxin, antihistamine, anti-viral among many other benefits. Most importantly, it helps regulate blood sugar and reduces depression and stress. High doses of Vitamin C can cure many illnesses. Vitamin E, on the other hand, is used to fight heart disease, for healing burns and also useful in treating epilepsy. I am neither a nutritionist nor do I hold a medical degree, but I have been through enough to know exactly what is lacking and what my body needs. I had been consistently sick for almost five years when I decided to learn everything I could about nutrition. Don't let this be the case for you. Rather choose *prevention over cure*!

In order to make a change and allow individuals such as yourself to know how to take care of your health properly, I wrote this book! Your physician will never tell you the truth about how to handle your body properly. They need your cash in order to survive! It all comes down to switching to natural foods. Your body cannot heal one thing and leave the other; therefore, one Vitamin cannot eradicate this lack. The body has its own healing mechanism to fight bacteria and viruses every day to keep your entire system in great shape. Studies have shown that the Mediterranean diet is the best one for a healthy weight loss as it contains the healthier fat, which lowers your risk of heart disease and other cardiovascular illnesses while increasing your life expectancy.

The Mediterranean diet is typically followed by the Greeks, Spanish, French, and Italians. This choice of eating includes healthy fats such as those found in avocados, olive oil, etc. It also includes plenty of vegetables, seafood, beans, high-fiber grains, and fruits. Fish and chicken are preferred over red meat, which is only consumed occasionally. It isn't really a diet, but rather a lifestyle. Eating meals of this type regularly can lead to a reduction of the bad cholesterol. Healthy eating does not have to rely on Mediterranean diet alone, cruciferous vegetables also can play a useful role in getting you healthy. Dark, leafy green vegetables, such as spinach, kale, and exotic lettuces, are packed with beneficial vitamins, minerals and other nutrients, as well as, being completely free of unhealthy ingredients. By incorporating them into a healthy diet, the savvy dieter will get plenty of healthy nutrition, mostly in the beta-carotene form, Vitamin A. Keep in mind that a low calorie diet is not the same thing as a balanced diet. It is possible to eat only carrot sticks every day and you will have a low-calorie diet, yet it will be a horrible diet nutritionally speaking. To keep your diet healthy, you should try to consume as many fruits and vegetables each day as possible. A daily allowance of fruits and veggies combined is roughly 9-19 servings a day. That sounds like a lot, but it is really not difficult to fit them in. A simple way to increase the amount of vitamins and minerals in your diet is to increase your consumption of vegetable juice. Juices are full of vitamins and nutrients and are healthy alternatives to sodas. When you combine Vitamin C with foods containing iron, the two nutrients are absorbed more easily. Spice things up by mixing things together like ginger, bananas or grapes. You can even have half a jalapeno for a good spicy taste. Refer to the juicing recipes in Section 2.

More views will be changed when more and more people become aware of the bad effects of unhealthy foods and habits. A very stressful life for example, pushes the body to break down more of the Vitamin C and a lack of it might cause vulnerability in your cardiovascular system and a weakening of your immune system in the process. The root cause of many diseases is lack of vitamins. A cardiovascular disease is considered to be a disease of civilization and lifetime because we are eating too much of the wrong thing. Vitamin A can be found in yellow, pumpkin, orange, and dark green vegetables such as kale, Bok Choy, collard green, spinach and many other cruciferous nutrients. The nutrition found in these delicious vegetables can boost your immune system by neutralizing the free radicals that attack the healthy cells. To improve a poor appetite, try snacking on foods that contain zinc. A zinc deficiency has been proven to decrease your sense of taste and lower your appetite. Zinc-rich snack foods include pumpkin seeds, yogurt, and peanuts. Turn to the nutritious pumpkin seeds instead of eating junk food when you get a craving. These snacks are extremely delicious and can help curb your appetite as well. Vitamin C can be found in almost all vegetables and fruits, including strawberries, tomatoes, broccoli, and mainly citrus fruits. It improves your overall energy to get you going during the day instead of relying on high calories and chemically induced energy drinks. There are various vegetables that one can add to his or her diet. Some of those important vegetables include:

Spinach

Spinach is a common and inexpensive vegetable that can be found around the world. This particular vegetable best grows in cool weather, which is where most of its taste comes from. Spinach is rich in nutrients and minerals, especially magnesium, which supports bones, muscles, and nerve health; calcium which is good for bones and assists in teeth reconstruction; and potassium, which is important for cell health. Spinach also has a good amount of iron (essential for the proper functioning of red blood cells). It can help maintain vision, reduce blood clotting, and strengthen bones.

How to Incorporate Spinach into Your Diet

Spinach can be used in various ways. It can be:

- Added to soups, stews, salads, pasta etc.
- Sautéed to pair with meat, fish and other seafood dishes.

- Juiced alone or along with other fruits and vegetables.
- Used in smoothies as well as omelets, sandwiches, cakes, etc.
- Used to make dips.

Raised Concerns

Due to the high amounts of pesticides used in the production of crops, especially in the United States, it is necessary to wash your spinach thoroughly before using to avoid any contamination including the free radicals in your body. To be safe, get your spinach from an organic provider and avoid those from supermarkets or look for the label "organic" before purchasing. Furthermore, in case you suffer from kidney stones, stay clear of spinach among other foods and use kale or other substitutes instead. Last but not least, always consume your spinach with a Vitamin C supplement to ease the absorption of iron and calcium found in the vegetable. The possibilities are endless when it comes to a vegetable with broad versatility such as spinach. Spinach can also be alternated with kale for a great energy boost.

Tomatoes

Tomatoes can be considered as a functional food. They can be added to any meal or be eaten as a fruit. They provide basic nutritional needs and provide additional properties in the prevention of chronic disease, while delivering other health benefits. An important nutrient in tomato is chlorine, which is known to help with muscle movements, sleep, and learning and memory. It also helps maintain the structure of cellular membranes which aids in the transmission of nerve impulses, assists in fat absorption and reduce chronic inflammatory problems. A healthy consumption of tomatoes helps with hydration while regulating your bowel movements due to its high water content. Tomatoes also can help combat the formation of cancer cells due its richness in Vitamin C and other important antioxidants which also clean out free radicals from your body.

Nightshade tomatoes have pros and cons nutritionally. Consider them carefully. They may not agree with your digestion. On the other hand, they may add real food value to your diet. They are easy to add because they are naturally sweet, and attractively bright without added artificial colors. They are also very versatile, as they can be eaten raw out of hand for more nutritional value.

How to Incorporate Tomatoes into Your Diet

Tomatoes have to come from a natural source to reap the benefits listed above. Pesticides and other chemicals are widely used by mass production farms, consequently sacrificing the taste and the nutrients of the food. Above all, tomatoes have to be stored at room temperature to retain their flavors and their redness. The consumption of ketchup does not replace your tomato consumption. Ketchup is full of sugar and preservatives, which are causes of diabetes, some cancers and obesity. The possibilities are endless when it comes to tomatoes. It is up to you to use them as you please.

Tomatoes can be:

- Added to stews and soups.
- Added to avocados for a tastier guacamole.
- Added to salsa.
- Added to hummus or dips
- Added to salads, sandwiches, omelets, rice, tacos, quesadillas, etc.
- Eating fresh as a fruit or can used to make bruschetta or other appetizers.

Kale

A cup of kale a day, keeps the doctor away! The leafy green vegetable is packed with maximum nutrition putting it on top of the ANDI (Aggregate Nutrient Density Index) chart. Even spinach does not come close to comparing with kale. Leafy green vegetables such as kale are rich in iron, vitamins and minerals. They promote the overall health of hair, skin and nails, bone health and protein, and improves one's blood pressure, controls glucose (especially for diabetics), and lowers the risk of asthma development. The essential nutrients that kale contains are: vitamins A, C (more than 1000% of daily recommended intake per cup) and K as well as minerals including iron, manganese, copper, potassium, phosphorous and protein.

How to Incorporate Tomatoes into Your Diet

Kale, along with other vegetables, is known for their versatility and low calorie content. Because kale is a typical lettuce that is healthy and crisp, it has many uses. Kale can be:

- Sautéed with a hint of olive oil, garlic, and other seasonings, to be accompanied with seafood or meat.
- Used for salad as it grows more in the winter months to replace Romaine lettuce or spinach in your dishes.
- Added to soups, stews, sandwiches, wraps, casseroles, and many other dishes you find fitting.
- Juiced or added to smoothies.

Carrots

We were always instructed by our parents to eat our carrots; unfortunately, we lost those values when we grew up. Carrots, which come in various shades of orange (the most popular), red, purple, and yellow, are usually found in farmers' markets. The shade of the carrot is based on the variety of antioxidants it contains. Carrots are naturally sweet and crunchy with a bright orange color. A single carrot is loaded with exceptional nutritional content adding more to our dietary needs. Just like many other vegetables, carrots are rich in magnesium, vitamin E, zinc, manganese, phosphorous, folate, potassium, vitamin K and fiber. Carrots are important in reducing the formation of cancer cells. A deficiency in Vitamin A can have damaging effects on one's vision which is why the consumption of beta-carotene rich foods such as carrots is important in vision restoration and improvement.

How to Incorporate Carrots into Your Diet

Incorporating carrots into your diet doesn't have to be a hard task. They are a versatile vegetable just as kale, spinach, etc.

- Carrots can be eaten raw, steamed (better than cooked), boiled, and added to many dishes such as: soups, salads, stews, and vegetable juices for flavor.
- Love baking? Avoid adding sugar! There are so many other options that you can use to make your cake just as tasty. You can substitute half of the unnecessary sugar with carrot juice. They can be as tasty as real sugar. This also adds the extra benefit of getting extra fruits and vegetables in your diet.
- Prepared in breads and muffins with different vegetables. Be sure to use a recipe that is low in fat and sugar. Eating bread or muffins with carrots in them is a good way to add more natural nutrients to the diet.

Collard Greens

Each time a new season rolls around, a new crop of healthy, nutritious veggies appears just waiting to be enjoyed. Collard, beet, mustard, and turnip greens have greater nutritional values loaded with illness fighting components such as Vitamin C, calcium, beta-carotene, and fiber. Just as other vegetables, collard greens provide fewer calories and fill stomachs faster due to its fiber content along with other glorious vitamins it contains. Collard greens come with loaded calcium. Most of us were taught that dairy products are the only way of satisfying our calcium needs. Animal dairy products are loaded with illnesses, leaving us at the mercy of medicines, while collard greens are loaded with vitamins necessary for our survival.

How to Incorporate Collard Greens into Your Diet

Store your greens in a well-chilled environment or they will become bitter. To keep vegetables fresh longer, be sure to wrap them in a damp paper towel and then put them in an airtight plastic bag. Greens should be used within 3-5 days. T

- Collard green can be served with meat or seafood.
- They also can be added to your stir-fry for optimum flavor and health benefits.

Mustard Greens

Mustard greens have been consumed for more than 5,000 years. It originated in the Himalayas, a region of India. Mustard greens just as turnip greens are widely used in different cuisines ranging from Asia to South America. Mustard greens have the ability to bind bile acids in the digestive tract when consumed frequently. They also act as an anti-inflammatory which helps detoxify the body system. As an impeccable sources of Vitamin C, E A (carotenoids), K and manganese, mustard greens provide a higher level of support to our dietary supplements. Mustard greens also has cholesterol-lowering abilities.

How to Incorporate Mustard Greens into Your Diet

- Mustard greens should be purchased from an organic, local source to reduce your pesticides intake.
- They should be not be blemished, and should be free form any yellowing or browning spots. They should be bright with green with healthy leaves.
- They should be rinsed thoroughly with cold running water and be individually halved before usage.
- If not cooking the greens right away, sprinkle them with lemon juice before letting them sit to induce more flavor and available nutrients.
- Mustard greens should be sautéed to be added to soups, stews, fish or meat.
- Great additions to pasta dishes or in combinations with pine nuts, goat cheese, or other chopped vegetables.

Bok Choy

Bok Choy means "soup spoon," deriving its name due to its large shape. This vegetable is popular among Asians. Its leaves resemble collard greens while its stalk is as smooth and white as romaine lettuce. It grows to reach about 12-18 inches in length. This entire vegetable can be used in various ways. The leaves can be used in soups and stews and the stalks can be used in salads or in stir-fry to release their best flavor. This dish will make you forget the taste of fried foods! Not only is Bok Choy a versatile vegetable, it is also loaded with cancer-fighting abilities along with other health benefits that are still to be discovered. Bok Choy is generally low in calories, and also comes loaded with calcium. magnesium and vitamin K.

How to Incorporate Bok Choy into Your Diet

Although Bok Choy is produced year round, it is best to consume it during the wintery months. Most of us get sick from the dry air and the cool weather it brings, thus with Bok Choy, it is easier to heal your body and reinforce your weakened immune system.

- Always buy fresh and organic vegetables. Avoid purchasing those with witted and lusterless leaves.
- Store them in the fruits and vegetables compartments of your refrigerator. Humidity is essential for its storage.
- Consume Bok Choy within 3-5 days of purchase to preserve its nutrients, sweetness and flavor.
- Trim the base and remove the outer discolored leaves, then wash it with running cold water later, pat it dry or place it down to drain out all the water.
- To prepare, separate the outer stalks and equally halve them using a knife.
- Chop the stem end about an inch apart and work your way towards the leaves.
- You can sauté them with garlic, a dash of olive oil, salt and pepper to serve with other dishes.
- The stalks and leaves are great additions to stir fry, rice, cabbage coleslaw, poultry, fish etc.

Cauliflower and Broccoli

Broccoli and cauliflower are packed with essential nutrients and vitamins. They are known as nutrient-dense foods in that have a high dose of nutritional value in a small amount per servings. Both are cruciferous vegetables. A cup of broccoli contains about 220% of the Vitamin C you need each day, as does a 3.5 ounce serving of cauliflower. About one-sixth of a head of broccoli provides you with 100 percent of your daily recommendations. Broccoli contains iron, Vitamin A, potassium, and calcium, while cauliflower is a good source of Vitamin C. Recently, studies have identified various advantages of broccoli consumption. Broccoli may:

- Help fight osteoarthritis.
- Protect and prevent skin cancer and delays the aging of skin.
- Increases the promotion of enzymes that help protect your heart blood vessels, reversing your risk of heart disease.
- Reduce your risk of developing cancer.

Cabbage

Cabbage is tasty when eaten raw, but many vegetables are palatable only when cooked. It is a good idea to add cabbage to your diet. Not only does it store well, and is a versatile ingredient in everything from burgers to the humble coleslaw, but it's filled with copious amounts of fiber, Vitamin C, Vitamin K, and lots of minerals. It also helps in bone synthesis. The humble cabbage family provides us with an especially good buy, nutritionally. Cabbage is very versatile. It can be fermented, chopped to be added to soups and several dishes.

Romaine Lettuce

Romaine lettuce is known for its Vitamin C and beta-carotene content, which is highly beneficial to the heart's proper function and the prevention of heart attacks. Lettuce contains fiber, which helps keep your digestive system in great shape. Fiber is known for reducing future cravings and helps in lowering the cholesterol level in one's body. Romaine lettuce contains folic acid. Folic acid is known for helping the heart, just like Vitamin C and the beta-carotene. This lettuce is also rich in potassium, which helps reduce your blood pressure, decreasing your risk of heart disease. Romaine lettuce is also known for its high water content and low caloric count. It is also rich in vitamins (B1, B2, K, A, and C), chromium, folate, manganese, and other minerals (molybdenum, iron, phosphorus, and potassium.

Onions and Garlic

Things that we often neglect are the ones that add the most value to our health. Apart from adding flavor, onions and garlic have many beneficial health values, including vitamins and minerals. Studies show that garlic lowers blood cholesterol, and triglycerides, as well as blood pressure. Garlic consumption may lower your risk for certain types of cancers, heart disease, high blood pressure, and high cholesterol, just like the consumption of onions. You can increase the beneficial compounds in garlic by letting it sit about 15 minutes at room temperature after chopping or crushing it before you cook it.

Onions, on the other hand contain essential nutrients like quercetin, a flavonoid that may lower your risk for cancer, heart disease, and cataracts. Onions can help you meet your recommended intake for fiber, potassium, Vitamin B6, folate, and Vitamin C. The best way to consume them is by including them in your meals, especially breakfast.

Parsley and Cilantro

Parsley and cilantro are great additions to your meals, and both belong to the *apiaceae* family. Parsley leaves are used for medical treatment and a variety of culinary purposes. Cilantro, sometimes known as coriander, has similar uses as parsley, and also plays a great role in mercury (which is usually found in fish) elimination. It also makes a great addition to your daily juicing and adds a great flavor to it. Cilantro has a more delicate appearance than parsley, but both offer a variety of nutritional values. Parsley contains a variety of nutrients such as Vitamins A, and C, folic acid, and iron. This vegetable is very flavorful, makes a great decoration for food, and is abundant in minerals. Some of the well-known benefits of parsley are its magnesium, calcium, potassium, and zinc. This vegetable also contains a huge amount of fiber and is known to reverse the cancer-causing effects of fried foods or high-carbohydrate diets.

Parsley comes with some added benefits which are the following:

- It helps eliminate excess water from your system (promoting weight loss).
- It eases diarrhea.
- It eliminates bad breath after a meal.
- It helps to regulate menstruation cycles.
- It purifies the blood and dissolves cholesterol.

Cilantro reduces bad cholesterol, in the body. In some cases, cilantro is known to de-stress the body just by smelling it or drinking it in a liquid state.

Some of the advantages of cilantro are:

- It acts as an expectorant.
- It helps ease conjunctivitis, as well as eye-aging, macular degeneration, and other stressors on the eyes.
- It contains immune-boosting properties.
- It reduces minor swelling.
- It helps in fighting anemia.

Be aware of adding these two vegetables in oil as it may lessen their effectiveness and add unnecessary calories into your diet. Read on to learn further.

Food Alternatives and Oils

Gradually replace your unhealthy habits with healthy ones. Many mistakenly eliminate foods that they enjoy, which tempt them to go off track. Beware of salad dressing that contains a ton of sugar and fat. You could make your own dressing with vinegar, with healthier oil like bran oil, flax-seed oil, or olive oil. Be wary of using too much olive oil; make sure you sprinkle it instead of pouring. Although it is very nutritious, it is quite high in fat. The less oil you ingest, the less fat you put on your thighs. Do your best to swap high-calorie foods with similar low-calorie alternatives; for instance, use low-fat yogurt instead of puddings or custards, or use vinegar on your salad instead of buying a vegetable dressing such as ranch. The recommended vinegars to use are: wine, white, balsamic, rice, etc. Find the taste that most suits your needs and stick to it.

Learn to enjoy healthy foods and increase your chances of success. As previously stated, color plays a great role in choosing vegetables for healthy nutrition: the darker the color, the better the nutritional values. If there is something really unhealthy that you just absolutely enjoy, find a good substitute. For example, for people who love white pasta, there is a great substitute made from squash. When you put sauce on top, it becomes almost impossible to notice the difference from real pasta.

Substitute slices of fresh raw vegetables for potato chips. Sometimes, when you have the munchies, nothing will do except something crunchy. Potato chips are not a healthy choice! Slice up some celery, squash, zucchini, cucumber, or whatever other crunchy vegetables you can find in your fridge. Add some low-calorie homemade salad dressing, and bon appétit!

If you have a child who is a picky eater and you are worried that he or she isn't getting enough nutrition, try hiding vegetables in other foods. Use pumpkin or zucchini in muffins, or puree carrots and apples in a pasta sauce. There are lots of ways to sneak fruits and vegetables into snack foods for your child. The beginning will be difficult, but as you move along, it becomes easier to welcome the changes in your lifestyle. Flax-seed oil is excellent for someone who wants to drop inches. Hence, use it in your vinegar salad dressing to transform your meal from ordinary to extraordinary! Here is a small chart of different oils you use with their calories and nutrients contents:

Note: All nutritional information in this and other charts throughout this work are taken from the United States Department of Agriculture (USDA) Agricultural Research Service (http://ndb.nal.usda.gov/ndb/)

Oils

Food	Portion	Cals	Calci	Sugar	Potas	Sod	Prot	Fat	Fiber	Carb	Sat Fat	Vit C
Almond oil	1 tsp.	40	—	0	—	—	0	5	0	0	0.4	—
Avocado oil	1 tsp.	40	—	0	—	—	0	5	0	0	0.5	—
Butter oil	1 tbsp.	112	—	0	—	—	0	13	0	0	8	—
Canola oil	1 tbsp.	124	—	0	—	—	0	14	0	0	2	—
Coconut oil	1 tbsp.	117	—	0	—	—	0	14	0	0	12	—
Corn oil	1 tbsp.	120	—	0	—	—	0	14	0	0	2	—
Cottonseed oil	1 tbsp.	120	—	0	—	—	0	14	0	0	4	—
Grape seed oil	1 tbsp.	120	—	0	—	—	0	14	0	0	1	—
Hazelnut oil	1 tbsp.	120	—	0	—	—	0	14	0	0	1	—
Olive oil	1 tbsp.	119	<1g	0	—	<1g	0	14	0	0	2	—

Palm oil	1 tbsp.	120	< 1g	0	——	< 1g	0	14	0	0	7	——
Peanut oil	1 tbsp.	119	——	0	——	0	0	14	0	0	2	——
Shea nut oil	1 tbsp.	120	——	0	——	0	0	14	0	0	6	——
Sunflower oil	1 tbsp.	120	——	0	——	0	0	14	0	0	1	——
Soybean oil	1 tbsp.	120	——	0	——	0	0	14	0	0	2	——
Vegetable oil	1 tbsp.	120	——	0	——	0	0	14	0	0	2	——
Walnut oil	1 tbsp.	120	——	0	——	0	0	14	0	0	1	——

Weight loss involves tips and tricks in order to make the process much easier. There are no magic pills to shred the pounds overnight. Only knowledge, patience, and hard work will determine your success. Weight loss should no longer be a struggle for you. Losing weight can happen and it is easily feasible. Follow these tips and you will have no trouble losing the extra weight that you have been trying to shred for years. To broaden your understanding of fruits and vegetables, I have put together a list of some of the nutrients found in vegetables including their caloric counts. I hope you find it useful!

Vegetable Chart

Food	Portion	Cals	Calci	Sugar	Potas	Sodium	Prot	Fat	Fiber	Carb	Vit C
Asparagus (spears cooked)	½ cup	23	19	—	208	347	3	1	2	3	22
Arugula (Fresh)	½ cup	3	16	—	37	3	<1g	<1g	<1g	<1g	2
Fresh Artichoke (Cooked)	1 med	60	54	—	425	114	4	<1g	7	13	12
Basil (Freshly Chopped)	2 tbsp.	1	8	—	24	0	<1g	<1g	<1g	<1g	1
Bay Leaf (Crumbled)	1 tsp.	2	5	—	3	<1g	<1g	<1g	<1g	<1g	<1g
Beets	Sliced or whole	35	0	5	—	290	1	0	2	8	2
Cooked plain Beans	½ cup	180	64	—	376	504	6	1	6	26	4

Food	Serving										
Broccoli (Spears cooked)	½ cup	25	127	—	166	22	3	<1g	3	5	37
French Beans (Dried and cooked)	1 cup	228	111	—	655	11	12	1	17	43	2
Red Beans (Dried Cooked)	½ cup or (4.6 oz.)	90	20	3	—	560	6	0	5	20	0
Black-eye Peas (Organic)	½ cup	90	30	1	210	25	7	1	4	16	0
Carrots (Sliced)	½ cup	17	19	—	131	176	<1g	<1g	1	4	2
Cauliflower (Cooked)	½ cup or 2.2 oz.	14	10	—	88	9	1	<1g	1	3	28
Celery (Raw Diced)	½ cup or 2.2 oz.	10	24	—	172	52	<1g	<1g	1	2	4
Fresh Cilantro	1 cup	11	31	—	235	25	1	<1g	1	2	1
Cloves (Ground)	1 tsp.	7	14	—	23	5	<1g	<1g	—	—	2

Food	Serving										
Coriander (Fresh Leaf)	¼ cup	1	4	—	22	1	1	<1g	<1g	—	<1g
Yellow Corn	½ cup	66	—	—	—	—	2	1	1	15	—
Chickpeas (Canned)	1 cup	285	78	—	413	718	12	3	<1g	54	9
Eggplant (cubed and cooked)	1 cup	28	6	1	246	3	1	<1g	3	7	1
Garlic (Freshly chopped)	1 tsp.	4	5	<1g	11	0	<1g	<1g	1	<1g	1
Leeks (Chopped and Cooked)	¼ cup	8	8	—	23	3	<1g	<1g	—	2	1
Lentils (Dried and Cooked)	1 cup	231	37	—	731	4	18	1	—	40	3
Mushroom (Pieces)	½ cup	19	—	—	—	1	<1g	—	—	6	13
Mushrooms (chanterelle)	3.5 oz.	12	5	155	165	1	1	<1g	6	13	3

Food	Serving										
Okra (Sliced and cooked)	½ cup	25	50	—	257	4	1	<1g	—	6	13
Olives Tapenade	1 tbsp.	25	20	1	—	210	0	3	0	1	2
Onions Chopped	½ cup	21	51	—	124	416	1	<1g	—	5	—
Pickles (Low Sodium)	2.3 oz.	12	6	—	75	<1g	<1g	<1g	1	3	1
Rhubarb (Fresh)	½ cup	13	52	—	175	2	1	<1g	—	3	5
Sweet Potatoes (Mashed)	½ cup	172	35	—	301	21	3	<1g	3	40	28
White Beans (Dried &Cooked)	1 cup	249	161	—	1003	11	45	1	—	45	0
Wild rice (Cooked)	1 cup	166	5	—	166	5	7	1	3	35	0

Fruits and Nutrition Tips

Calories is often an underused word when discussing dietary contents. Many popular diets prioritize specific food groups over the overall picture, leading many to overeat and sit dumbfounded and full. To help you add more nutrition to your diet, savor the flavor of seasonal fruits and vegetables. Whether you grow them in your garden or purchase them from a local farmers' market or a convenient, neighborhood supermarket, vegetables and fruits that are in season provide maximum flavor and nutrition. They are also easy on your wallet! Fill at least half your plate with fruits and vegetables, and eat them first.

Since these will be the healthiest things on your plate, you should start by eating your vegetables. You may feel yourself getting full before you move on to your less healthy foods, which can help you get the best nutrition possible. Focus on healthy foods that will provide you with the vitamins and nutrients your body needs. Fruits, vegetables, legumes, nuts, and whole grains are excellent sources of nutrients and should comprise the majority of your diet. Make these foods a regular part of your menu and you will get plenty of fiber, calcium, Vitamin D, and potassium.

Fruits are the best food when discussing healthy eating, as they are sweet and easy to move around with. Fruits are naturally sweet, with a low glycemic index scale score, as well as in terms of calories and fat. Fruits also provide powerful antioxidants, and essential vitamins and minerals, and best of all, they fill the stomach quickly due to their water content. Some fruits, when consumed alternatively, promote healthy weight loss compared to ice cream or cakes for dessert.

Below are some of the fruits that contain the maximum nutrition you need daily. Put them to great use, and you will notice a significant change.

<u>Bananas</u>

Bananas are a staple for a no-fuss snack or breakfast in the morning. They are the fruit we most consider for our morning smoothies, and snacks.

They are perfect due to their great packaging and cause no mess when it comes to carrying them along for work, school or on a trip. They are a little higher in calories than most fruits that we use in our daily nutrition. Apart from their great taste, bananas are great for individuals struggling with their weight. They are low on the glycemic index and provide us with the daily strength that we need to tackle our day ahead. Bananas offer carbohydrates to the body most importantly, in Vitamin C, B6, fiber, potassium, and minerals.

A single serving of a banana provides about 30% of the recommended daily amount of B6. We have previously discussed this vitamin, but to refresh your memory, Vitamin B6 is a great component in helping keep the immune system at its peak, and a lack of it could cause some risky damages to one's body.

How to Incorporate Bananas into Your Diet

Bananas are a wonderful, natural energy bar. They contain a great deal of natural sugars to give you an immediate pick-me-up, but also have potassium for stamina and recovery after a workout. Also eating a small snack before working out (about 30-60 minutes before you start exercising). A good example of a pick-me-up before a workout would be a banana along with a low-fat yogurt, or oatmeal sprinkled on top. You will have energy for your workout and will not be distracted by hunger pains. Replace your high-sugar, meal-replacement bars or energy bars with a banana.

Feed your children healthy snacks with bananas. Ignore those pre-packaged sugary snacks, and introduce your children to healthy snacks disguised as fun treats! Something you can do is dip a banana in vanilla yogurt, then roll it in crushed cereal, and freeze. Another tip is to spread frozen yogurt on two graham crackers and fill them with sliced bananas to make a tasty 'sandwich'. Mix cornflakes with peanut butter, roll into balls, and cover with crushed graham crackers. Slap some peaches, apples, pineapples, bananas, and other fruit on the grill and get ready for a real treat. Fresh fruit such as a banana makes a wonderful addition to a backyard cookout.

You don't have to eat it raw every time though! You can cook it right alongside the lean hamburger and turkey franks!

Kiwi

Kiwi is a green fruit with a brown skin. This fruit that we all love to gobble for breakfast or snack is one of the healthiest fruits due to its fiber. It contains high amounts of vitamins and minerals, with reduced amounts of calories and fat. The availability of these nutrients promotes proper balance for great cell function, regular nerve response, collagen production, proper communication of neurotransmitters, immune system health, and proper blood clotting.

How to Incorporate Kiwi into Your Diet

You can consume your kiwifruit through juicing, fruit salads, and many other dishes for a healthy meal. Get your kiwi organically (pesticide-reduced or free) or through your local farms at a cheaper price compared to the ones you get from your supermarket.

Berries

Berries such as boysenberries, blueberries, raspberries, cranberries, and strawberries are among the best things that you can eat during the course of the day. They contain 10 times the antioxidants levels compared to other fruits. Berries also contain nutrients such as folate, copper, manganese, magnesium, potassium, and riboflavin. Anthocyanin, Vitamin C and quercetin are powerful antioxidants found in berries. Anthocyanin, for instance, is responsible for the vibrant color in berries. Its objective is to reduce inflammation and could prevent arthritis. Anthocyanin works with quercetin to slow down memory loss, which is accompanied with aging. Quercetin reduces the inflammation effects in the joint, especially for health conditions such as rheumatoid arthritis.

Berries are generally full of water and make a great addition for weight loss since they fill you up quickly and are low in calories. The volume observed from berries comes from water, fiber and folate. Folate protects against aging-related memory loss and cardiovascular disease whereas fiber and water aid in weight loss while lowering your bad cholesterol levels and decrease your blood pressure. Folate also contributes to the production of serotonin, which is responsible in lifting depression while improving your mood swings.

How to Incorporate Berries into Your Diet

- For a healthy breakfast, you can make a smoothie with a mixture of berries. They are very versatile and are natural boosters for a great morning. A simple recipe is to pour a cup of fresh fruits such strawberries, blueberries or any other fruits in a blender along with four ice cubes, milk and two or three tablespoons of yogurt depending on the thickness you desire. You also can add a teaspoon of honey to improve the taste.
- In addition to making fruit smoothies with berries, you can also add fruits to foods your kids already enjoy. Try topping pancakes with strawberries and blueberries instead of syrup.
- In case you want a nutritious treat that your children would enjoy, make caterpillar kabobs. Cut fruits such as fresh pineapple, oranges, melon, apples, and strawberries into bite-size chunks. Assemble the chunks of the colorful fruit on a skewer to form a fruity caterpillar kabob. Since the fruit is on a skewer, monitor young children when they are eating this treat.
- With the same berries, you can make your dessert healthy, too. Instead of chocolate cake, try raspberries dipped in chocolate. Instead of ice cream bars, opt for homemade ice cream with real strawberries. Remember that healthy foods don't have to be boring, and they can be very tasty!

Oranges

An orange is a delicious, nutritious, and refreshing fruit that should be considered instead of coffee. It provides enough stamina to kick your day off with a great start and contains multiple vitamins and minerals that are necessary for a healthy body, especially its antioxidant content, which contributes to a healthy immune system.

One orange gives about 140% of the RDA (Recommended Daily Amount) of Vitamin C. The sweet taste alone pushes kids to consume it more often, which is why it is recommended that you juice it yourself instead of purchasing the packaged juice, which might contain way too much sugar for your child's body.

Oranges are also rich in potassium, which is responsible for muscle health, as it makes them work better and at the same time prevents high blood pressure.

Pears

Pears can be a great addition to salads, juicing, and many other uses. Eating pears entails many benefits, including helping with digestive distress, muscle cramping, body hydration, and some illness prevention. Pears are a wonderful source of nutrients. They are durable and sweet, and come in a variety of textures, including creamy, juicy, and crunchy. They have lots of fiber and potassium. Pears are rich in water, which ranges from 83 percent to 88 percent. As you might be aware, hydration is known to help muscles recover rapidly from injuries and helps the body recover rapidly from illnesses. This fruit is versatile and can be used in most of our foods. Pears are rich in fiber and potassium. A delicious, quick snack can be a puree of berries, pears, or other fruits. Pureeing these fruits results in a paste that makes a good topping or dip for many different foods, from chips to pretzels.

Summary

Now that you know a little more about nutrition, you can see that it's not very difficult to stay properly nourished. There are many foods out there with great health benefits and many ways to help you stay as healthy as possible. The key is simply making a few changes to tweak your appetite for healthy foods. Caloric count and the awareness of the nutrients founds in the food we consume give us a broader aspect about what is healthy to consume and what's not. The chart below contains some of the well-known fruits we consume daily. Now you will be able to know how many calories it has and how much to consume!

Fruits Chart

Food	Portion	Cals	Calci	Sugar	Potas	Sodium	Prot	Fat	Fiber	Carb	Vit C
Apples (Fresh)	1 Med	81	10	——	159	1	<1g	<1g	4	21	8
Avocado (Mashed)	1 cup	407	25	——	1458	28	5	40	11	16	18
Apricot (Halved with Skin)	1 cup	65	19	——	465	7	2	<1g	——	16	8
Banana (Fresh)	1 med	109	7	——	467	1	1	<1g	3	28	11
Blackberries (Fresh)	½ cup	37	23	——	147	0	1	<1g	3	9	15
Blueberries (Fresh)	1 cup	82	9	——	129	9	1	1	——	20	19
Cantaloupe (Freshly Cubed)	1 cup	57	17	——	494	14	13	<1g	1	22	68
Cherries (Sweet and Fresh)	10 pieces	49	10	——	152	0	1	1	——	11	5

Food	Serving										
Grapefruit (Water Packed)	½ cup	44	18	—	161	2	1	—		11	27
Grapes (Fresh)	10	36	5	—	93	1	<1g	<1g		9	5
Honeydew (Freshly Cubed)	1 cup	60	10	—	461	17	1	<1g		16	42
Melon (Frozen Balls)	1 Cup	55	17	—	484	53	1	<1g		14	11
Mulberries	1 Cup	61	55	—	271	14	2	—		14	51
Orange (Florida)	1 Whole	69	65	—	254	1	1	<1g	4	17	68
Papaya (Fresh Cubed)	1 Cup	54	33	—	359	4	1	<1g		14	87
Passion Fruit (Purple Fresh)	1 Whole	18	2	—	63	5	<1g	<1g		4	5
Peaches (Halves Water packed)	1 Half	18	2	—	76	3	<1g	<1g		5	2

Pear (Halved Water Packed)	1 Half	22	—	5	41	<1g	<1g	6	1
Pineapple Sliced (Water Packed)	1 Slice	19	9	74	1	<1g	<1g	5	5
Raspberries (Fresh)	1 Cup	61	27	187	0	1	1	14	31
Strawberries (Fresh)	1 Cup	45	21	247	2	1	1	4	10	85

For the best nutrition possible, eat foods that are still close to their original form. Fresh food that has not been processed will help you take care of the nutritional needs of your body and drive those unwanted chemicals and fat out of your system. Dairy products are great sources of calcium and Vitamin D, which helps to build bone mass. Make simple meals that your family will love! If your refrigerator is stocked with nutritious ingredients such as the ones mentioned above, you can ensure that those you love will always have access to healthy foods. Keep in mind that nutritious foods are useless unless eaten. If you are proactively mindful about eating better, your whole family will have better nutrition.

Effects of Processed Foods and the Chemicals Used in Making Them

Bad food can cause serious health-related issues not only for the brain, but also for the rest of the body. We should take care of our bodies more often by fueling them with good ingredients rather than consuming foods that help dig our graves one shovel at a time. I have been a victim of this sensation, but there are many dangers involved long after your moment of enjoyment has passed. Many cigarette smokers have tried tirelessly to abandon their nicotine consumption in vain; rather, they found themselves wanting more and more cigarettes. This issue has been a concern in American society for years. Therefore, if fatty foods (snacks and beverages) have the same effects as the nicotine thrill, the consumer's battle for safety is put into question. Obesity in America is growing day by day due to the availability of the processed food that surrounds us. Whether at work or on the road, we always find those hydrogenated oily processed chips to cope with. Many have battled those processed foods' manufacturers, but changes are barely noticeable; it is up to us to take a stand and demand better or healthier products. Nowadays, our hospitals are filled with aching patients with dangerous illnesses, and it all started with a bag of chips or a diet cola! Below are some of the chemicals used in the production of foods in the United States:

Aspartame

Aspartame is by far the most dangerous chemical added in food. Aspartame is one of the most thoroughly studied food ingredients ever. Consumer research shows that low-and reduced-calorie foods and beverages have become part of the lifestyle of millions of men and women who want to stay in better overall health, control their weight, or simply enjoy the many low-or reduced-calorie products available. This drug is the real cause of obesity and fatal diseases such as cardiovascular disease.

Saccharin

Saccharin is an artificial sweetener component that is mostly used to reduce the consumption of regular sugar. It is commonly sold under the names Sweet'N Low or Sweet Thing. Saccharin is approximately 300-500 times sweeter than regular sugar, and its side effects are costly, including: Headaches, stomachaches, high blood pressure, vision issues and many others. Remember that each body is different from the next, and we each show different side effects towards a product. Be cautious about what you put in your body, and if you have to have a sweetener for your beverage, please use it in a low or moderate quantities.

Sodium nitrite

This substance is found in some foods and is capable of being converted to nitrous acid when ingested by humans. It is still being used by our food industry, which strives for profit rather than quality.

Nitrates and nitrites

These two chemicals are used to preserve red and white meats such as ham and bacon. They are known to cause asthma, nausea, vomiting, and headaches in some individuals, but their use continues.

Sulfur dioxide

This toxin is used in dried fruits and molasses, as well as to prevent brown spots on peeled fresh foods such as potatoes and apples. This chemical basically bleaches out rot, hiding inferior fruits and vegetables. During food processing, this toxin destroys Vitamin B contained in produce, making it empty or limited in nutritional value.

Benzoic acid (sodium benzoate)

Whenever you pay attention to your food labeling, you will notice that this toxin is added into your margarine, fruit juices, and carbonated beverages. It is known to produce severe allergic reaction and in severe cases, death.

MSG (monosodium glutamate)

Glutamate is a flavor enhancer that is widely used in bottled products, fast foods, and spices. Glutamates were discovered in Germany in 1866, and their use quickly became a global practice. This chemical is extracted from sodium salt of glutamic acid, which is where the name comes from. The chemical is naturally addictive and is widely used by many food companies. It is also found in crackers and many cheese-flavored chips. MSG causes weight gain and asthma attacks, exacerbates migraine headaches, causes throat swelling in some cases, chest pain, and malnutrition, as many consume it for their taste buds rather than for valuable nutrition. Pay attention to any food you purchase and only purchase those with "no MSG added" on the label.

The Cost to Society

Each time you turn on your television, you notice celebrities with slim bodies, promoting cheap foods for Americans to buy. We are constantly bombarded by advertisements misleading us that we can become thin by using their various products for a shorter period of time. There is an idea that weight can be magically lost without any major effort involved. Health costs from obesity in America is rising each year! Weight gain is a lifestyle choice and can be eradicated by consuming the right foods. The cost to society is enormous when it comes to processed foods. Obesity causes several dangers, such as: heart diseases, sleep apnea, strokes, diabetes, and some cancers in severe cases. Many businesses and individuals are now coming to grips with these problems because of the cost of health insurance, which has burdened their wallets. The non-obese often must bear the cost of the obese. Obesity is slowly becoming a monumental issue that is often discussed by policymakers as well as those in the private sectors seeking to mobilize and find solutions for this epidemic disease. There have been endless campaigns criticizing the higher costs of obesity and the various diseases it brings about. Most kids have been overweight their whole lives and find it very difficult to let go of their old habits. The food companies are mostly the ones to blame for obesity, and most of their advertisements are directed to children who tend to get their foods outside of their homes. By teaching these children about healthy eating at an early age, they will be much more likely to turn to better eating options in their adulthood.

The ecological health is not considered when it comes to the food industry's earnings! Most food manufacturing employees are basically treated like human machines. Sadly, most of them are undocumented, saving the industry owners billions of dollars since they are under no strict rules of giving workers' compensation rewards. After the invention of the fast-food restaurant, things turned worse, causing high negligence of the workers with no benefits.

Basic Steps to Reverse Our Actions

Choose foods that are in season, buy foods that are organic, and read the labels! The average food travels 1,500 miles from the farm to the supermarket; hence, purchasing foods that are grown locally not only sustains your community's economy, but it stretches your dollar and helps you consume pesticide-free or pesticide-reduced items. Make a habit of cooking a meal together with your family and have family dinners regularly. Everyone has the right to healthy food! Make sure your farmers market takes food stamps. Ask your school board to provide healthy school lunches. You can make a difference by changing every bite you consume. Now that you are aware of what it takes to produce your food, let's work on repairing the damages caused by your old eating habits!

Benefits of Detoxification and Juicing

Our body naturally detoxifies itself every day as part of a normal body process. Unfortunately, body systems and organs that were once capable of cleaning out unwanted substances inside our tissues are overwhelmed with unwanted chemicals. A good cleansing diet can revitalize your system and get rid of harmful bacteria, viruses, and parasites from one's body. The colon, lungs, liver, lymph nodes, kidneys, and skin mainly ease detoxification and neutralize toxins to allow the body to properly function. With the pollution found in the air, water, and food we eat, our bodies have a hard time keeping up. Our chemically rich diet with too much bad protein, saturated fats, trans fats, caffeine, and alcohol radically changes our internal system. Detoxification through special cleansing diets and colonics is the best way to assist your body's natural self-cleaning system and repair cells that have been damaged by your bad diet. The process of detoxification cleans out toxins and many other unwelcome chemicals from the intestines and organs. There are thousands of ways to eliminate bad chemicals from the body, however the two most well-known, effective and safest forms of detoxification are: Raw Vegetable Cleansing and Colon Hydrotherapy.

Raw vegetable cleansing can be done daily and can be varied to avoid redundancy and boredom. This type of cleansing usually comes in the form of a supplement containing minerals-derived soluble, insoluble fiber and vitamins that a body needs in order to clean itself properly. Additionally, it assists your body in cleansing the colon of accumulated toxic build-up and impacted fecal matter and helps prevent the formation of new build-up if continued daily or weekly. It is more effective when combined with seeds such as chia seeds and flaxseed. Here are some seeds to include in your diet and their nutritional content:

Food	Portion	Cals	Calci	Sugar	Potas	Sodium	Prot	Fat	Fiber	Carb	Vit C
Sunflower Seeds (Dried)	1 Cup	82	168	—	992	4	33	71	—	27	—
Squash Seed Roasted with or without Salt	1 oz.	148	12	—	229	5	9	12	—	4	—
Organic Flaxseed	¼ Cup	140	—	0	—	0	5	9	6	10	—
Pumpkin Seeds (Dried)	1 oz.	154	12	—	229	5	7	13	—	5	—
Sesame Seeds	1 tsp.	16	4	—	1	1	1	2	<1g	<1g	—

The most important vegetables one should include in the diet are the ones with higher ANDI score. Kale is one of the vegetables with a high nutrient density and can be easily versatile. Fruits and vegetables can be added to give the juicing more taste. The most common fruits to add are apples, bananas and pineapples. These three fruits give more taste to your juices and give them an appealing color, especially when feeding it to children.

The second method is called *Colon Hydrotherapy*. It is a safe and effective method of removing waste from the large intestine, without the use of drugs, and most importantly, it assists in weight loss. It is a simple three-step process which is done via a disposable speculum which is then introduced into your bowels. The whole process is done with filtered and regulated temperature water to soften and loosen the feces, resulting in waste evacuation down through disposal waste tubing that is attached to a colon therapy machine. This therapeutic process is then repeated to gather other wastes that were bypassed. You can visit the nearest colon hydrotherapy center to learn more.

As you eat healthier, your risk of cancer or diabetes slows down and reinforces the cells in your body to promote a healthy body, reducing your trips to the doctor's office. The foods that include most of the proteins and other necessary vitamins are fruits and vegetables. Some of the jumbo vegetables contain fewer calories than half a steak. The best vegetables to consume are the green vegetables due to their richness in antioxidants and minimal calories and fat and their richness in chlorophyll. No matter your consumption of carrots, kale and many great vegetables, you will still lose your weight and enjoy a healthy life. You need to consume high nutrient foods to balance your good nutrition. Eating healthy increases your chances for weight loss and make you feel lighter after each meal.

Chapter Three

The Art of Organic Cooking

Eating well and taking supplemental vitamins are the keys to maintaining one's health. For you to appreciate what *Eating Smartly* means, you must understand that having a well-balanced diet is very simple, but also very important for your physical and mental well-being. The human body requires the proper mix of vitamins, minerals, proteins, fats, and carbohydrates in order to function. Food is fuel for any living being, and having a good understanding of what is good for one's body is important. Lean meats, fruits, vegetables, and grains are all crucial for one's daily diet. An Egyptian proverb stated that "about one quarter of what we you eat keeps you alive. The other three quarters keeps your doctors alive." This results from high processed foods that give us a great amount of pleasures leading us into the "pleasure mood". Drug usage is comparable to bad eating in a way that it triggers the brain to desire more and more, causing diseases and weight issues, leading you to a dietary survival mode. Most crippling diseases found in America can be reduced or simply eradicated by a simple and cost-effective system called the "Whole Foods plant based diet". It is based on consumption of foods that are minimally refined such as grains, fruits, vegetables, and legumes while avoiding or reducing animal foods such eggs, meats and dairy as well as processed foods like refined sugars, bleached flour, and oil. Whole plant-based foods are much healthier than animal-based foods. When consuming a typical Western diet, you lose most of the defense system which is important as you age. Eating more Whole Foods related foods will stop fatigue throughout your day and reduce your risk of diseases.

Many of us find ourselves feeling a little down during the cold, dark winter months, but eating certain foods can help to improve our mood. To see results, you should consume at least four cups of fruits and vegetables per day, as well as whole grains. This will help to raise serotonin levels (Omega-3 fatty acids, found in certain fish, olive oil and flaxseed can help enhance your mood). Additionally, avoid all forms of caffeine, as this decreases serotonin levels. Ascorbic acid, also known as Vitamin C, is crucial to keep in your diet. It is used for the maintenance of multiple body systems. It is found in many popular fruits and vegetables, but it is also sometimes added to foods as a preservative. For better nutrition, consider eating your fresh fruits and raw vegetables. Not only is it easier for your body to break down foods in their original state, but raw produce contains many vitamins, minerals, and other nutrients that steaming, boiling, and frying removes. It is also a good decision to eat the skin of the fruit or vegetable, if possible, as most of the nutrients are near the surface. When it comes to sports, nutrition is very important, and it must be well planned to match with the training program you have in place. A vegetarian diet would be best, emphasizing foods from the legumes, grains, and fruits and vegetables groups. Choose foods from these groups and focus on wholesome foods rather than processed. Research the various nutritional and health benefits of fruits and vegetables. This way, it will be uncomplicated to incorporate a mix into your diet that helps as preventative measures, as well as nutritional. The prolonged health benefits of the right choices in nutrition are as important as what is needed to meet the daily requirements of the body.

Juicing needs to be the base on which you grow your entire healthy lifestyle and weight loss. Make it a point of having juice every day to start you off with energy, nutrients, and a tasty breakfast. When it comes to juicing, one thing that you want to keep in mind is that it is a good idea to stock up on a variety of different fruits and vegetables. This is good because it will help ensure that you do not become tired of a certain taste. Juicing may seem very difficult, but if you take the time to learn about it, you will find that it can be done quickly and easily. This is a great way to provide your children with all of the nutrients that they need in order to grow up healthy. Juicing helps lower your cholesterol levels in a safe and medicine-free manner. It is great for treating acne from the inside out. Foods like apricots, carrots, grapefruit, pumpkins, strawberries, and watercress, all include the best vitamins and nutrients to battle the causes of acne. They are also taste great, and so they are far more enjoyable to treat your skin than chemical creams. Make sure to be tested regularly and stay under the care of a medical professional while attempting juicing for a treatment for cardiovascular diseases. The best produce to use include the following: apples, blueberries, garlic, kale, kiwi, because they include the most nutrients needed to reduce bad cholesterol in the blood. It's especially important to learn about necessary juicing equipment. Before purchasing a juicer, mixer, or blender, read some consumer reviews and focus on the ratings. Find a product of good quality so that it can suit your needs.

Here are great tips to get you started:

- Keep your juicing regimen simple. If you make it too complicated, you'll be less likely to stick with it.
- Instead of using elaborate juicing recipes with several different types of produce, just stick with two to three vegetables.
- Coconut is a natural way to enhance the sweetness and overall flavor of your mixture. Even if you do not care for the taste of coconut, you can try adding small amounts to give you good results, good taste, and good texture.
- Apples blend nicely with many different vegetables and lend a bit of sweetness to each recipe.
- When coming up with a combination of fruits or vegetables for juicing, consider their textures to make a smooth, drinkable product. For example, soft fruits like bananas and peaches make a very thick juice. Apples and pears, on the other hand, make a very thin, watery juice. Mix the two items together to make the most enjoyable texture to drink.
- Leafy vegetables have a strong taste and may be too much for you to start with on their own.
- Jerusalem artichokes are an excellent addition to the juice you make as they will kill any craving your sweet tooth throws at you. Since they are not as flavorful, add other items like lemon and carrot juice to make a drink that you'll enjoy and that will keep you healthy.

Juicing is the best way to get your children their vegetables. You can juice some fruits and vegetables together to create a great taste and keep children in the dark about the vegetables that they are drinking. One great way to get kids involved in juicing is by having them pick the fruits and vegetables you use! You can take them to a farm to choose their own apples, or to a farmers' market. The child can wash the produce while the adult chops it. Don't ever criticize them for choosing the wrong item; just use less of it so no one will notice.

Men and women of all ages benefit from nutritional principles, but this is especially true for children. You need to educate your children about healthy foods so that they grow into healthy eating habits that will follow them into their adulthood. On the other hand, if children eat lots of unhealthy foods containing sugar and fat, they will probably feel lethargic and may experience more growth stunts than they would have had otherwise. Children naturally want to be involved in whatever their parents are doing. Thus, it is smart to get the kids involved in making healthy dishes, making school lunches, and preparing nutritious snacks.

This is a golden opportunity to teach your children to make healthy decisions, which will follow them throughout their adulthood. When you do your shopping, give your kids a chance to choose some of the foods. If they have a choice in the vegetables purchased, they will be more inclined to consume them. This simple trick also pushes young children to eat new things when they are able to pick out the condiments that appeal to them most. You can also take them for family outings on a farm to observe the growing of food. Let them enjoy the environment! If it is summer-time, grow food with them and let them be in on the process by giving them each a chore. Growing food together as a family increases your chance of getting your children to eat better and healthier even if you are not looking.

Shelled unsalted sunflower seeds, flax-seeds, and pumpkin seeds are excellent options to try. You can even include cooked grains. Making healthy juice from vegetables is wonderful; however, do not go overboard with variety. Stick to using two or three vegetables in your juice blends and incorporate apple into the mix. You will minimize the amount of flavors you are trying to combine, and the apple will add the right amount of sweetness to the mix for extra enjoyment. It is important to clean your juicer as soon as possible after you are finished juicing your produce. The small bits of the juice remaining will become sticky if left in the machine for extended periods of time. If you do not have time to completely clean the appliance, at least give it a thorough rinse. A great juicing tip is to wash your juicer in the dishwasher. This is a great way to clean your juicer without having to exert much effort. Some juicers specifically state that you shouldn't wash them in the dishwasher, though, so you should pay close attention to the manual.

Juicing should be added to your daily lifestyle to increase your well-being. Once you have learned a little about juicing, you will find that you will be able to make great juices with no problems and eliminate the free radicals from your body. Juicing is one of the easiest and most natural ways to boost your nutrition intake.

If you choose to use the tips presented, you can now begin juicing with your favorite fruits and vegetables to produce amazingly healthy and tasty beverages. If you have reached a point where you have run out of new ideas, go to the nearest bookstore and find cookbooks of recipes, or look online. Keep your interest high by alternating old favorites with new exciting combinations. Becoming a juicing expert can make you healthier, help you lose weight, and give you plenty of delicious drinks to enjoy.

If you rely on juicing as your morning "wake-me-up", you will surely get through your day and suppress your hunger! Do not use extremely sweet fruits when juicing. The juices may taste better than others, but their sugar will raise the level of your blood sugar, which can contribute to a harmful effect to your body. Add in some vegetables instead to create a healthier juice option. It is okay to add in a piece of really sweet fruit, every once in a while, as a special treat, but on the whole, it is best to avoid them!

If you can't afford to juice with organic fruits and vegetables, don't worry about it. It's nice to have pesticide-free items, but you can only work with what you have available. Wash your produce in a mixture of eight cups of water with three tablespoons of hydrogen peroxide and three tablespoons of baking soda to get all the nasty stuff off. Rinse your produce well before using. Do not leave out vegetables from your regular diet just because you are getting them in your juice. Even fresh juice from the supermarket does not provide all of the same benefits as eating whole vegetables, especially when it comes to fiber.

Creating a healthy juicing habit is going to be easier if you keep your juicing machine out on your kitchen counter and in open sight at all times. When you know that you are going to juice on a particular day, try to set your vegetables out at least a few hours before using them. You want the vegetables to be room temperature because using cold vegetables for juicing can irritate your digestive system and cause numerous different stomach ailments. One option to remind you of your juicing is to set up a small area in your kitchen with your cutting board, peeler, knives, and favorite cups so it is easier to get fresh juice when you are passing through the kitchen.

In case you're very deficient in a vitamin like B12 and can't find it in the fruit and vegetables you're juicing with, add in some powder! Grind up your recommended dose and put it into your juice, making it easier to swallow and digest. Be careful with the medicines you might be putting in as some can react to various fruit, like grapefruit, and you could end up with a dose that is too potent, making it inadvisable to consume. Do not take extreme measures in order to benefit from juicing fasts. In fact, a fasting plan that is less extreme is more practical and feasible. For instance, replace one meal of the day with fresh fruit and vegetable drinks, or you might do a 24-hour juicing fast every 5-10 days. Fasting is a topic that general medicine and health professionals are generally undecided about. Short juice fasts are a way to give the body a boost and a break without embarking on a fasting diet that may be too harsh or restrictive for your body and or nutritional needs, and a 24-hour juice detox can be a great way to jumpstart a diet, but it's important to accompany it with a healthy eating plan that you can naturally fall into once the fasting day is over.

When juicing for weight loss, it is important to eat the pulp, as it contains a lot of fiber and nutrients that you need. Mix it with non-fat, unsweetened yogurt for an excellent breakfast item or after-meal dessert treat! You can mix it with non-fat yogurt, or actually pour it into your glass of juice. It is very important to drink the juice as soon as possible while it is fresh. This will ensure that you are receiving the maximum benefits. Some nutrients begin to be destroyed right away through oxidation. If drinking immediately is impossible, you can store the juice in an airtight container and drink within 24 hours.

If you don't want to drink vegetables, don't. Juicing doesn't have to freak you out every time you throw something into the machine! Start with things you know you don't mind drinking, like oranges and apples or even carrots. The money saved and the knowledge of what really is in your drink is what makes juicing so awesome! Refer to my detox recipes to get a jump start on juicing! As always, talk to your doctor before starting any kind of detox diet.

Chapter Four

Beverages

Water and High Water Content Foods

While we are advised to consume eight glasses of water daily, there are many more benefits of water than many of us are aware of. Your saliva, digestion, absorption, circulation, transportation of nutrients, and maintenance of body temperature all depend on water and it is up to you to help your body with the amount of fluids that it requires to maintain your organs and your body in good health, including your skin! Whenever you are low in fluids, your brain automatically activates the thirst alert, pushing you to consume water. Most tend to replace water with sugary drinks which unfortunately is transformed into fat by your pancreas. Water has no calories or fat! It is easier to be processed by your body, and excreted quickly compared to heavy dishes and soft drinks. For years, many dieters used water to lose their weight instead of eating real food, which can hurt your body as well. Healthy and well-functioning organs need healthy fat and calories to function properly and get you through your days. While water is not a magic potion to immediate weight loss, it is essential for our bodies and is far more useful compared to high-calorie beverages like colas. The most effective way to lose weight is the substitution of high-caloric beverages with no caloric beverages, or consumption of higher water content foods such as watermelon to provide the body the satisfaction needed. Water-rich foods include fruits, vegetables, broth-based soups, some legumes, and breakfast meals like oatmeal.

Some of the benefits of more water consumption include:

- **Helps Prevent Muscle Injuries**

  The thirst after a rugged workout is the result of a decrease of fluids, which shrivel due to muscle fatigue. Whenever a lack arises, the muscles refrain from delivering the performance which causes dizziness, weakness and sometimes fainting in some severe cases. Water is the most important beverage of all. Scientists recommend roughly 17 ounces of fluids two hours before exercising. This gives the body ample time to digest the liquid and distribute it to the organs and muscles to prevent injuries. Sweating is normal! Seeing sweat means the body is working and keeping you in a great shape. The mechanism of sweat is there to reduce toxins from the body, leaving it healthy and functioning at an impeccable rate.

- **Healthy Skin**

  The secret to longer-lasting skin is water! Dehydration makes the skin dry and dull, especially during summer. The skin needs plenty of water to function properly as a protective barrier to prevent premature aging and dull-looking skin. Be careful of over hydrating yourself. Everything is done gradually and on a continuous basis! Once your skin is adequately hydrated, your organs, including your kidneys, take over and excrete the excess fluids out, including the harmful toxins. To accelerate the glow of your skin, dermatologists recommend the consumption of more water and frequent moisturizing, especially during the wintry months.

- **Kidney Health**

  The main toxin that is excreted through urine is blood urea nitrogen. An adequate amount of water in the body helps with the excretion of waste, leaving the organs and the overall body functioning healthily. Water is mostly excreted through urine after it passes through the kidneys. The kidneys' role is to clean and get rid of toxins, and as long as you consume adequate amounts of fluid, (water) more chemicals will be excreted, leaving you with a stronger and healthier body.

- **Healthy Bowel Function**

  An adequate amount of liquid helps prevent constipation. Whenever you do not get enough fluid, the colon gets its liquid from the stools to maintain hydration, and as a result, you get constipated. A healthy body should include a recommended amount of water to ensure healthy hydration of your fiber, which acts as a vacuum to keep your bowel healthy.

In order to shed weight, you should avoid any sugary beverages. If you must, it should be consumed in small amounts as these drinks are packed with more calories than you might think. A healthy consumption of water is the following: About nine cups per day for women and roughly 13 cups for men. There are always exceptions to this recommendation, but keep in mind that these figures are just a rough estimate. Water is essential for weight loss and if used appropriately, you could lose more weight than you anticipated. Follow the tips below and put them to great use:

- Drinking a glass of water will prevent you from feeling hungry, which will result in you not eating too much. In addition, water helps your digestion and helps to regulate your body's hunger pattern. Not only does water help you slim down; drinking a good amount of water can flush the body of potentially harmful toxins that can leave your skin feeling oily.
- In case you find it difficult to just drink plain water, you can mix it with a lemon, a cucumber slice, or some other citric fruit to dress up the ordinary beverage, or drink green tea. Green tea can contribute to improving your nutrition.
- In order to get your system started out right every day, squeeze lemon juice into a cup of warm water and consume it. The citric acid in the lemon stimulates your stomach to produce the acids

necessary to digest food. The more efficiently your stomach works, the more nutrients it can get from your food.

Sugar's Effect

Americans consume way more sugar, especially teenagers. For a while, I thought avoiding carbs and exercising were the best forms of weight reduction but I was stunned after reading about the effects of sugar in our body. Sugar is known as a "fat producing hormone" and it is the most dangerous of all foods one could consume. We drink soda and other sweetened beverages thinking it will helps keep us in balance with our weight or give us the weight we desire sadly; we end up causing more harm to our bodies than eating fatty foods. We add sugar in our coffee, lattes, teas, and lemonade and the worst part is we even feed it to children, who get addicted to the pleasurable taste. An increased consumption of sugar decreases the level of vitamins and minerals in the body. Consuming less sugar decreases your risk of cardiovascular diseases. Eating less than 10% of calories from sugar as recommended by WHO (World Health Organization) pushes you to a step further to a healthy start. Below is an equation to help with your daily sugar consumption based on a 2,000 caloric diet.

Remember that 10% of sugar is recommended daily therefore multiply it by 2,000 which is the daily caloric input to find the right amount then divide the number by four calories to find the daily amount of calories to be consumed.

To limit your sugar consumption, you have to choose foods that contain natural sugars such as: cereals, fruits, vegetables, milk and plain yogurt. Not only do these foods limit your sugar consumption, but they are also packed with vitamins and minerals. Candy, soda, ice cream, artificial energy drinks, cookies, cakes, sweets, syrups and many other "man-made foods" or "junk food" are loaded with sugar and should be avoided at all cost. As you might have noticed, there are various benefits involving a healthy consumption of water. The best way to consume water is during your meals and during and after your physical exercises. Choose beverages that are low in calories, and eat more fruits and vegetables to promote good health. Last but not least, keep a bottle of water with you to enjoy during your thirsty periods. Having a bottle of water with you will decrease the likeliness of high caloric intake. It is much better for your health when you control what goes into your body. So, try some of these ideas that you have read, and you will be well on your way to enhancing your health. Below are many types of sugar and their nutrient contents:

Type of Sugar	Portion	Cals	Calci	Sugar	Potas	Sodium	Prot	Fat	Fiber	Carb	Vit C
Brown Packed	1 Cup (7.7 oz.)	828	167	214	762	86	0	0	——	214	0
Brown Unpacked	1 Cup (5.1 oz.)	546	123	——	502	57	0	0	——	141	0
Maple	1 Piece (1oz.)	100	26	——	78	3	0	< 1g	——	26	0
Powdered Sugar	1 tbsp. (0.3 oz.	31	0	8	0	0	0	0	——	8	0
Sugarcane Stem	3 oz.	54	2	——	——	——	1	0	3	14	1
White	1 tsp. or 4 grams	15	0	4	0	0	0	0	——	4	0
White	1 packet (6 grams)	25	< 1g	——	< 1g	< 1g	0	0	——	6	0
White	1 cup or 7 oz.	773	2	200	3	3	0	0	——	200	0
White	1 tbsp.	45	< 1g	——	< 1g	< 1g	0	0	——	12	0

Alcohol

Stop drinking or at least cut back on alcoholic drinks while dieting. Beer has tons of carbohydrates, and the sweet drinks are full of sugars and other artificial sweeteners, which only stimulate your appetite. There are other alternatives to satisfy your alcoholic thirst. Alcohol is the worst part of any weight-loss program. On the other hand, alcohol like red wine has important health benefits, like antioxidants, but should not be addictive; only drink half a glass for lunch and dinner. Alcohol dehydrates the body, causing injuries and exhaustion. Beers and other brews have high amounts of calories and lie in your midsection and make it difficult to burn the calories. "Beer belly" is another nickname of the effects of brewed beer, which is why it should be a constant reminder.

A moderate consumption of alcohol has been associated with some health benefits; however, researchers have discovered that excess alcohol consumption could interfere with your fat-loss abilities. The consumption of alcohol causes cravings of more foods, which leads to greater calorie consumption depending on what is being ingested by the individual. Most individuals, especially men, mostly consume beer, whiskey, and various sorts of soft drinks. The safe amount recommended is one drink (1.5 ounces of hard liquor, 12 ounces of beer, or 5 ounces of wine) for women and a maximum of two drinks for men. Wine can be used to accompany our meal. Wine is mostly consumed with French and Mediterranean dishes. I suggest you choose red wine, as opposed to white wine. Compared to white wine, red wine has less sugar and healthier nutrients. Nutritionists believe that drinking one glass of red wine per day may increase your life expectancy. The same idea applies to dark chocolate. Red wine has 125 calories per 5-ounce serving, and the best part is its antioxidants, which protect against heart disease and help maintain healthy levels of cholesterol. Red wine is also beneficial for diabetics, as it reduces the levels of insulin in one's bloodstream. Drinking a glass or two per day can be beneficial for individuals with Type II diabetes. While red wine contains many health benefits, it is recommended to consume greater amount of water daily than alcohol. For a non-alcohol version of mulled wine, try mulled Concord grape juice. Use the same spices you would use for mulled wine, and add honey for extra sweetness if you desire. Keeping a pot of this delicious, nourishing drink warming on your stove through the winter to enjoy frequently. It will help you stay healthy thanks to the beneficial spices and the vitamins provided by the grape juice.

The chart below will give you a further understanding about water, other beverages sold on the market and some well-known liqueurs.

Food	Portion	Cals	Coffee	Sugar	Potas	Sodium	Prot	Fat	Fiber	Carb	Vit C
Coconut water	1 cup	46	58	—	600	252	2	<1g	—	9	6
Coffee (regular)	1 cup	4	5	1	64	5	<1g	0	0	1	0
Coffee (Decaffeinated)	1 cup	4	6	—	63	6	<1g	0	—	1	0
Chai Tea (Brewed)	1 cup	140	300	14	—	50	6	4	0	19	0
Diet cola	12 oz.	2	12	—	0	21	<1g	0	—	<1g	0
Gatorade (All Flavors)	1 cup (8 oz.)	50	—	14	30	110	0	0	—	14	—
Ginger ale	12 oz. can	124	12	—	5	25	<1g	0	0	32	0
Red Bull	1 can	110	—	27	—	200	0	0	—	28	—
Rockstar energy Drink	8 oz.	110	—	27	35	35	0	0	—	29	60

	Serving										
Tea (Brewed, Chamomile)	1 cup	2	5	0	21	2	0	<1g	0	<1g	0
Water (ice cubes)	3 ice cubes	0	1	—	0	2	0	0	—	0	0
Water	8 fl. oz.	0	—	0	0	0	0	0	—	0	—
XS (tropical energy drink)	1 can	8	—	0	25	24	2	0	0	0	0
Beer, Wine and Liqueur											
Beer (Light)	12 oz. can	100	18	—	64	10	<1g	0	0	5	0
Beer (Free alcohol)	7 fl. oz.	50	5	5	40	3	1	<1g	—	11	—
Beer (Regular)	12 oz. can	146	18	—	89	19	1	0	<1g	13	0
Chardonnay	4 fl. oz.	92	—	—	4	0	0	0	<1g	—	<1g

Champagne (Brut)	4 fl. oz.	84	—	4	0	0	4	—
Margarita	1 serving	173	—	3	0	0	11	—
Rum	1 serving (1.5 oz.)	97	0	1	0	0	0	0
Tequila	1 serving (1.5 oz.)	117	0	—	—	0	—	—
Vodka	1 serving (1.5 oz.)	97	0	0	0	0	0	0
Whiskey	1 serving (1.5 oz.)	105	0	1	0	0	< 1g	0

NB: Liqueurs have fewer calories whenever they are served without any other ingredients or additional alcohol.

Chapter Five

Proteins

Our current food system promotes obesity. Have you ever pondered where your meat comes from? Well in order to get the truth, you will have to travel back to the origin to find out. I recently visited some of those farms and the reality is completely different from what is shown in our supermarkets. In order to push their products off of the shelves, they picture a farmer with healthy cattle or birds but in reality, many chickens have never seen the light of the day. Chicken are now fully grown in about 39-49 days instead of 90-120. Chickens are not raised naturally. They are injected with growth hormones to speed up their exponential growth. The goal is to produce a food with a very small land, small overhead and at a very affordable price. Cows on the other hand, are created to eat grass, but the reason why they are fed corn is because corn makes them fat very quickly for slaughter and corn is very cheap to produce compared to growing natural green grass. In 1972, the FDA conducted approximately 50,000 food inspections and in 2006, the FDA conducted 9,164. In the 1970s, there were thousands of slaughterhouses in this country; now there are basically 13 slaughterhouses that are processing and controlling the majority of the beef that is being purchased in the United States. Unfortunately, we believe in and consume the products of the food industry which still makes them relevant in the marketplace. Have you ever heard someone say "Time is Money"? This theory is vastly applied by each one of us and it is the push behind the food industry. Antibiotics are injected into animals to strengthen their immune systems which we consequently consume causing us more illnesses that we can counts. After all, none of the manufacturers will budge for your medical bills or mourn after your death! A body can be fixed by a skillful physician, but it can never be the way God created it. An organ for example is harvested from one body to another. It cannot be regrown by your physician. When supporting the food industry, be aware that your body cannot be replaced, it can be healed, but at the cost of emptying your bank account. Food is now considered a "product". What is wrong with that system? In order to get the truth, you are craving for, befriend a farmer and the truth about how your meat is produced will be revealed. Most of them might not to avoid any potential lawsuits, but some will. Our race toward cheaper food has pushed our farmers to reduce their costs and grow our meats faster and easier than before. One strategy is to upscale their operation by using cheaper labor and unthinkable methods to operate on a mass scale mindset. This cost-effective method is causing us more harm than we might know. A package of ground beef, for example, can come from thousands of cows. It doesn't come from one cow as are you are taught to believe through their packaging.

Sustainable farms can produce minimal environment impacts with naturally good tasty meat we can enjoy. Since sustainable farmers are just a fraction of the "big picture", there are some challenges to bringing their meats and dairy to every household in America. In order for them to succeed in what they know how to do best, they will need your help and support.

I have encountered several individuals wishing to purchase expensive cars or gadgets, but hate spending money towards their healthy eating. Thousands of organic markets are available at your disposal. It is up to us to control our food consumption. It is also up to us to claim organic foods instead of the "synthetic". Farmers are out to serve the general public and they will always turn to the high demand in a crowd. Health is never for sale! I learned this motto the hard way. Always ask for wholesome foods and you will change how the food is manufactured. Most importantly, purchase your animal products from companies that treat their workers and animals with care and respect. Meat in general has its share of trouble when consumed irresponsibly but it shouldn't cause diseases such as E.coli. Consuming quality meats in limited amounts will save you money in the long run. Always "think long term instead of short term".

Proteins and Nutrition

Excess fat intake and poor nutritional choices may cause inadequate micronutrients (Vitamins B6, B12, C, E, copper, iron, zinc, and others) consumption in the body. Your protein-based diet does not have to come from animal products, as we have been taught, but it can come from vegetables sources. We have to desire a low-carb diet, not just certain food portions on the plate. When considering a diet that provides an adequate nutrition level, understand that not all healthy-sounding foods are as healthy as you might think. Depending on the cut, ground turkey may contain nearly as much fat as ground beef. When shopping for meats, always look for the lean or low-fat variants. Initially, the food industry was praised for using science to find a way to create inexpensive food and feed more people than possible. But with the rise of deficiencies and diseases, there is a new focus on nutrition, and people have begun to question how science has undermined it. A good healthy diet should include foods that are low in fat and high in protein. Proteins will keep you fuller for longer and also will help regulate your blood sugar levels. White meat is generally healthier than dark meat. Eat a well-balanced meal at least three times a day that includes a source of lean protein. Chicken, turkey, and other poultry are all foods that fulfill these requirements, but only if they are consumed without the skin.

Ideally, poultry is boiled, baked, broiled, or roasted, but never fried. By choosing leaner white meat, you can cut a great deal of saturated fat and unhealthy bulk out of your diet, while still retaining the protein found in all meats. This substitution promotes a healthy heart, while giving your muscles the nutrients they need to repair damage and grow. Include these white meats in dishes such as sandwiches, salads, stews, soups, and much more; in short, the possibilities are endless. This category includes fish, chicken, turkey, beans, and tofu or soy products for vegetarians. Substitute animal products with food such as: tofu, beans, or even textured vegetable protein (TVP). These can make a hearty, tasty addition to any meal. Seasoning is what makes these meals so flavorful, so be creative with your substitutes. You may find yourself surprised at how versatile they are! Furthermore, to improve the function of your liver, include plenty of tryptophan in your diet. Tryptophan is an amino acid that helps your body synthesizes various proteins. It is essential in the production of niacin, which boosts liver health. Foods rich in tryptophan include salmon, turkey, and watercress. Tryptophan can also reduce anxiety levels. Remember that everything is only good in moderation. A good vegetarian diet (whole plant food based) is associated with health benefits such as lower LDL, lower heart disease rate, lower rates of Type II diabetes, lower blood pressure, and fewer cardiovascular disease-related illnesses. The truth is that it can be quite difficult for a non-vegetarian to indulge in the avoidance of meats and dairy products all at once, which is why they need a calorie count in order to stay on the healthy side of the equation. I, for example, have tried numerous times to avoid meat but was always unsuccessful; therefore, I decided to adopt the theory of "vegetarian on the weekdays and non-vegetarian on the weekends." In terms of healthy eating and weight loss, your primary focus should be on Whole Foods, rather than meat. Whole plant foods such as fruits, vegetables, seeds, whole grains, nuts, and beans are associated with health benefits. With this kind of diet, you can add a small portion of meat as well if you find it difficult to part with your meat products. You should know that processed foods and animal products account for 90% of our calorie consumption. The typical American diet lacks important antioxidants, vitamins, minerals, fiber, and phytochemicals that should be the main focus for our nutrition. In case you are the kind of person who despises calorie counts, the recommended way is to embrace more of a whole-plant foods-based diet. I am not encouraging you to avoid meat altogether, but just a reduction will make a difference in your weight loss, nutritional health, and best of all, for your life expectancy. Our ancestors consumed more whole-plant foods than they did with meat, which is somehow the tradition that my mother carried on with us.

While vegetarianism is not for everyone, most people consume far too much meat, especially red meat. Red meat is very hard for your body to digest, and the average person usually has too large a portion on his or her plate. If you eat meat, stick with fish and white meat, and keep the portion to a smaller size. A healthy diet should also taste good! If you are struggling with new foods that you do not like, try something different and be creative. You can improve your overall nutrition by selecting the proper proteins. Protein is necessary for muscle and bone growth, but we can choose the leaner types of protein that are available. Skinless chicken and fish that are high in Omega-3 fatty acids can improve the overall nutrition of any diet.

Nutrition during pregnancy has special requirements to ensure that your baby is as healthy as possible. Focusing on iron-rich foods will make sure that your developing baby will have an adequate oxygen supply during development. Iron-rich foods can also help prevent premature delivery. Good sources of iron come from vegetables and fish. Something everyone should consider in regard to nutrition is to add fish-oil supplements to their diet. Fish oils contain essential Omega-3 fats not found in other meats. These fats have a lot of health-boosting properties, such as lowering cholesterol and reducing inflammation, so if you can't eat fish regularly, consider fish oil capsules. Do not forget plenty of fruits and vegetables in addition to your fish, as they are packed with essential vitamins and minerals.

Moreover, make sure you take care about your health as much as you can by buying organic foods instead of chemically treated condiments that constantly cause us more harm than good. Protein is an essential part of your diet, and seafood is very high in protein. The goal in nutrition, first and foremost, should be health! Nutrition is not about what size you want to be or what dress or suit you want to fit into. It is about great health! The golden rule is to avoid eating anything that has more than 4g of sugar per serving. This will save a lot of calories, and it is particularly helpful for you to follow this rule if you are diabetic. Be aware of the chemicals added in your food. This is generally why it is best to stick to natural produce, fresh proteins, and organically grown grains. You should avoid sugar and chemicals as you would hazardous products because they can slow down your metabolic rate and harm your body severely.

A healthy regimen is to increase the amount of vegetables and fruits that you eat every day; at least nine servings are recommended. This may seem difficult, but it is actually easy to pull off. Next, focus on getting a lot of protein throughout the week. You can choose between seafood, white meat (skinless), and vegetables. Eggs also contain a wealth of protein. Studies have found that eating one egg daily will not harm your health. The healthiest and most useful advice is to have a meatless day at least twice a week. Use shiitake mushrooms as filler in recipes that call for ground beef, or tofu for other compatible dishes. Studies show that mushrooms satisfy the appetite nearly as much as meat, probably because of the texture. Mushrooms are much healthier, contain lots of fiber, and could have certain nutrients that fight off cancer.

Protein and Weight Loss

As mentioned, the animal or bird is not the issue. It all depends on where the meat comes from on that particular animal or bird. Every animal has areas where it stores more fat, even chickens. In some areas of the chicken, such as the thighs, you will find more fat than the amount found in a beef rump roast and twice the fat of a pork tenderloin. Lean meat is recommended by dietitians for more success in weight loss or the prevention of unwanted diseases. Consume ground turkey rather than ground beef. Small substitutions will get the nutrients you need while reducing your fat intake.

It can be quite difficult to substitute your red meat with white; therefore, your best option would be to consider how much is really enough for your red-meat consumption. Large servings of red meat can really affect your health. So instead of the 12-ounce steak, reduce it to 3-6 ounces per week, and try alternating your white meat with seafood such as fish or shiitake mushrooms to provide further health benefits. In case money is problematic, fresh or dried fish make a great alternative. Understand that not all fat is bad and that there are some foods that can provide essential fats that your body needs. Consuming these suggested alternatives decreases your cravings for fatty foods like fried chicken and pizza. Foods that have good fats in them include nuts, certain fishes, and avocados. Focusing more on serving grilled fish, clams, or tuna is a great way to cut down on calories, while still having meals that contain protein. Seafood is more enjoyable, particularly in the summer, due to its freshness. Seafood, like salmon, tuna, or lobster, gives your body the protein it needs for very few calories. It makes a healthy lunch or dinner, so make an effort to increase the amount of seafood in your diet.

Do not make the mistake of believing that eating meat is the only way you can add protein into your diet. There are many foods that can be consumed to increase protein, and many of them contain less fat than meat. These foods include nuts, beans, tofu, and seafood. You should consume iron-rich foods such as almonds, lentils, seafood, or lean red meat as part of your diet. Some common symptoms to watch for are fatigue, dizziness, and shortness of breath. Iodine is a mineral that should be a part of any healthy diet. It is necessary for production of thyroid hormones, which control your energy metabolism. It also works to prevent goiters. You can get iodine from seafood, dairy products, iodized salt, and bread has been fortified with iodine. Cut down on red meat by serving more seafood weekly. You may love red meat, but eating it every day is not in your best interest when it comes to nutrition and weight loss.

How many Calories, and how much Saturated Fat and Cholesterol should I consume?

Carbohydrates, sugar, fat, cholesterol, fiber, calcium, sodium, potassium, vitamins and many other nutrients are needed by your body to function properly! Every food you enjoy has a different assortment in nutrients. Milk, for example, is rich in calcium; fruits and vegetables are high in fiber and vitamins, and meats have lots of proteins in them so do some vegetables. When served together, they give a balance meal to promote a healthy body weight and an optimum health.

Calories (cals)

Every time you eat, you take in calories. Whether it is a scoop of ice cream or an apple, it has calories. Fats, carbohydrates, and proteins all include calories and are mostly referring to macronutrients. Your amount of calories should be equal to the amount of calories burned or to be burned. This is the most accurate way of losing or maintaining your weight. Whenever you consume more calories than you can burn, your body reserves it for the future, which never comes since there is a large availability of food at our disposal. You will notice these excess calories on your thighs, your hips, and your waist, which are such tricky places to store fat.

Almost all the calories that are consumed from our usual "American Diet" mostly come from proteins, carbohydrates and fat. Even the healthiest food has calories therefore, whenever you deprive your body from calories, you end up weak and unable to perform at your best. You will mostly feel tiredness and sometimes headaches, which isn't the best way of reducing your body weight. The secret of losing weight is burning as many calories as you consume.

How much fat, cholesterol, saturated fat and sugar should I consume?

For a healthy weight, an individual should consume 20-30% of their total calories from fat, meaning if you consume 2,000 calories daily on a regular basis, your fat content should be between 400-700 calories. Dieters who are able to get at least 20% of their calories from fat found it easier to shed weight compared to those who do not.

Cholesterol (Chol)

Men in America consume about 330mg of cholesterol daily whereas women consume about 240mg a day. The National Cholesterol Education Program recommends a limit of 200mg of cholesterol a day whereas the America Heart Association recommends a maximum of 300mg per day. Always know that the less cholesterol, the better for your health!

As always, you should consult your physician and have your blood tested before adopting any new diet(s).

Saturated Fat (Sat Fat)

There is not any specific amount of saturated fat to be consumed daily. In order to stay healthy, the National Cholesterol Education Program recommends 7% of daily calories from sat fat. As always, have yourself tested by your physician before adjusting your sat fat intake.

Before we compute your amount of body fat, know that 1g of fat = 9 calories; therefore, to compute the amount of sat fat to consume daily; you multiply your amount of sat fat by 9 (the number of calories per of fat).

2,000 *calories* × 7 *percent saturated fat* = 140 *calories sat fat a day*

To find out the amount of sat fat to be consumed daily:

140 ÷ 9 *percent* = **15 grams sat fat daily**

Proteins and Cooking Tips

In the past, we were told by health experts that eating between meals was not good for weight loss. Nowadays we know that snacking on healthy foods can reduce hunger and fend off binges. The best foods to consume are protein-rich foods such as string cheese or a slice of lean chicken or turkey; even a spoon of peanut butter spread on an apple or celery is a good dish for a snack! Remember that the healthier proteins you consume, the easier it will be to lose that extra weight. Healthy proteins include seafood (fish, crab, shrimp, etc.), poultry (lean turkey and chicken), and beans (essential for vegetarians), lean beef, and dairy products such as low-fat cheese or milk, but choose your dairy products wisely.

Dairy products are necessary for a full diet, but can be high in fat. Soy and almond milk are healthy alternatives compare to animal dairy products. While healthy protein is expensive, it is an important part of your diet. Lean white meat, such as lean turkey or chicken, provides large amounts of protein while avoiding excess amounts of saturated fat and carbohydrates. When paired with healthy condiments such as vegetables, it makes a perfect meal.

Add some lean protein to your lunch, because this will sustain your energy throughout the rest of the day. Stick to whole wheat bread and go with lean meats such as tuna, chicken, or turkey. Also use light or fat-free condiments. In case you feel like having a hamburger, do it yourself! What you need to know is to use a lower-fat meat alternative instead. All you do is get your lean ground turkey, and add sage, rosemary, and thyme with a little bit of Worcestershire sauce and Dijon mustard.

Grill or bake it to remove even more fat, and enjoy it on a whole wheat bun! If you are watching your calorie intake but crave something tasty, throw together a pot of low-fat chicken soup. Soup is mostly enjoyable in the winter and fall weather due to its richness in nutrients that are useful for your body's health. Try chicken, turkey, carrots, brussel sprouts, squash, even a diced sweet potato for a shot of healthy fiber. Last but not least, always use a low-sodium broth to make your meal.

Avoid meats that are high in fat such as pastrami, and stay away from unhealthy condiments. For example, you could prepare a turkey salad sandwich using some multi-grain bread and vinegar dressing, or hummus. This will save you a lot of money too!

While making your own lunch is a great way to control portions and calorie intake, beware of preservatives and other bad things lurking in meats. Sticking to high-quality chicken, turkey, and other light meats will help you evade additives, fat, and strange preservatives. Avoiding preservatives is a helpful way to reduce toxin intake. Farmers' markets are the best places for purchasing pesticide-free products and at the same time save you more money for other needs.

To ensure that you always have some high-quality protein readily available, pick up some frozen boneless and skinless chicken breasts to keep in the freezer. They are easy to defrost in a covered skillet over low heat. Add some instant brown rice and fresh vegetables for an easy nutritious dinner. Learn different ways to cook some of your favorite foods in a healthier manner. You may love the taste of deep-fried chicken or fries, but your body does not. There are alternatives in cooking methods for foods to still provide the taste you love without all the calories. Try baking, roasting, steaming, and broiling as alternatives to frying. If you are looking to cut back on fat and oil intake, try marinating your meats without oil. A popular marinade for grilled chicken can be made with two cloves of garlic, pepper (quantity as desired), chopped onions and a cup of low-sodium soy sauce. It's a brilliant sweet glaze akin to teriyaki, and low-fat as well!

Seafood also has plenty of iron, which is important to your diet as well. Senior citizens looking to be as heart-healthy as possible can enjoy a Mediterranean diet. This way of eating includes healthy fats such as those found in olive oil, including plenty of vegetables, seafood, beans, high-fiber grains, and fruits.

The Mediterranean diet lowers the risk of heart disease because of the healthier fats it contains. Poultry and animal meat play a role in one's diet unless you are a vegetarian. However, it is important to limit your consumption of meat, especially red meat. Seafood is generally healthier and contains fewer calories. As you can see, it is easy to plan for optimum nutrition and excellent health with just a few basic ideas to keep you on the right track. Looking and feeling your best, no matter your age, is within your control. Start using the suggestions provided above for your best nutrition! I have listed some of the proteins that we consume daily with the calories and carbohydrates contents below.

Food	Portion	Cals	Calci	Chol	Potas	Sodium	Prot	Fat	Fiber	Carb	Vit C
Bass (freshwater raw)	3 oz.	97	68	58	303	59	16	3	—	0	—
Beef (chopped)	2 oz.	170	0	40	—	810	7	15	0	2	0
Raw ground beef (extra lean)	4 oz.	265	7	78	321	75	21	19	—	0	0
Bison (Roasted)	3 oz.	122	7	70	307	48	24	2	—	0	—
Chicken skinless (broiler/fryer)	1/2 breast	142	13	73	220	63	27	3	—	0	0
Clams (meat only)	3 oz.	126	78	—	534	95	22	2	—	4	—
Cod (Atlantic Fresh)	1 fillet	189	25	99	440	141	41	2	—	0	2
Crabs (cooked Alaskan king)	3 oz.	82	50	45	222	911	16	1	—	0	—
Duck (Roosted with skin)	1 cup (4.9 oz.)	281	17	125	353	91	33	16	0	0	0

Food	Serving										
Roasted goat	3 oz.	122	15	64	344	73	23	3	0	0	—
Roasted goose without skin	6.6 oz.	574	25	172	618	132	47	41	0	0	0
Guinea hen (without skin)	1/2 Hen (9.3 oz.)	292	—	166	—	—	55	7	0	—	—
Lamb (cubed, lean and broiled)	3 oz.	158	11	77	285	65	24	6	0	—	—
Lobsters (cooked)	1 cup	142	88	104	510	551	30	1	2	—	—
Cooked Mackerel (Atlantic)	3 oz.	223	13	64	341	71	20	15	0	0	< 1g
Octopus (Fresh and steamed)	3 oz.	140	90	82	—	—	25	2	4	—	—
Oysters (steamed)	3 oz.	138	14	—	257	180	16	4	8	—	—

Lean Pork (ribs country style)	3 oz.	252	25	74	—	50	20	18	0	0	1
Salmon (Pink with bones)	3 oz.	118	181	—	277	471	17	5	—	0	0
Scallops (raw)	3 oz.	75	21	28	274	137	14	1	—	2	—

Section Two

During the process of writing this book, I have had the chance to interview some individuals who find it easier to have a weight-loss book with some suggested recipes. This section is mainly about Mediterranean, French, healthy recipes and celebratory drinks. It includes smoothies, soups, salads, several dishes, and lastly some delicious desserts you can enjoy with your family. Most of them are made with affordable ingredients so they could be used by a wide range of readers such as yourself.

Glossary

Bake: To cook in the oven until dry.

Beat: To use a fork, whisk or electric mixer to add air to a mixture in order to make it more voluminous, light, and creamy.

Blanche: To cook vegetables in boiling water for a few minutes.

Blend: To combine ingredients evenly to create one regular consistency.

Bouquet garni: A mixture of herbs such as thyme, basil, parsley and rosemary, tied together in a small bouquet with cooking twine and used to flavor sauces, stews, and stocks.

Braise: To slow cook and tenderize meat, fish, or vegetables with herbs and seasoning in either stock or wine.

Caramelize: To cook foods containing sugar or mixed with sugar over a low heat until melted in a golden color.

Chop: To cut into small pieces using a knife.

Coat: To cover something in a substance such as melted chocolate or breadcrumbs.

Color: To brown meat in a frying pan or pot over a hot flame.

Decant: To pour a liquid gently, normally wine; boil before transferring it to another dish.

Dice: To cut into small cubes.

Dress: To trim off the inedible parts of a food.

Fillet: To remove the bones from a fish using a small knife with a pointed blade.

Grate: To cut into fine shreds using a grater. It is usually done to some vegetables and cheese.

Grill: To cook on a wire rack under a direct source of heat.

Grind: To reduce a rough ingredient into powder using a mill, mortar, pestle or blender.

Ice: To cool a food or drink using ice cubes.

Infuse: To leave a length of time, often over a low heat, to extract the flavor.

Julienne: To cut a fruit or a vegetable into fine batons or sticks.

Marinate: To bathe meat, fish or vegetables in a rich sauce for a lengthy period of time to tenderize and to flavor.

Poach: To cook in liquid.

Reduce: To cook over a low heat to thicken and concentrate the flavor of a sauce.

Roast: To cook meat or a vegetable in the oven in an uncovered dish.

sauté: To fry briskly in a small amount of fat or grease.

Simmer: To keep a liquid just below boiling point.

Steam: Slowly cook something with the lid on using a small amount of liquid usually water.

Sweat: To cook vegetables in fat or grease without browning them for a small amount of time.

Whip: To beat with a whisk or mixer to incorporate air in order to add volume to a food mostly done with eggs.

Zest: To remove the tangy outer skin from a fruit using a peeler or a zester knife.

Chapter Six

Recipes

Smoothies

In order to have a healthy body, it is important to have a daily breakfast. It improves your cognitive skills and provides the necessary energy needed throughout the day. Studies show that people who eat breakfast tend to eat less during the day. In your breakfast, increase the amount of fruits you're eating by making a "breakfast smoothie". Smoothies are great, especially for kids! It is a way to hide traces of healthy ingredients that won't be visible to your children. Below are some healthy recipes for you to try!

Orange-Banana Smoothie

Oranges are full of Vitamin C. It is the favorite of our mothers, especially in the morning. When included in your smoothie recipes, it does wonders and wakes you up like a cup of coffee, but without the caffeine.

Preparation time
5 minutes

Cooking time
None

Servings
2 servings

Ingredients

- 1 cup freshly squeezed orange juice
- 1 banana
- 1 tsp. honey
- 3/4 cup low-fat milk
- 2 tbsp. yogurt
- 4 ice cubes

Preparation

Step 1: Wash your fruits if necessary and blend all the ingredients in your blender.

Step 2: Serve immediately.

Avocado-Berry smoothie

To eat a nutritious diet while suffering from an ulcer, look for soft, vitamin-rich foods that are easy to digest. Avocado is easy on a sensitive stomach, and is also full of fiber and healthy fats, which can help speed your recovery. This smoothie will ensure that you get those healthy nutrients that your body requires.

Preparation time
5 minutes

Cooking time
None

Servings
2 servings

Ingredients

- 1 cup freshly squeezed orange juice
- 1/2 avocado
- 8 strawberries
- 1/2 cup raspberries
- 1 kiwi
- 1/2 banana
- 6 ice cubes

Preparation

Step 1: Blend all the ingredients in your blender and add 1/2 tsp. of honey if not as sweet as preferred.

Step 2: Serve immediately.

Strawberry Smoothie

Strawberry is well-known as a fruit that assists in the prevention or reduction of acne. Consume it as often as you can to see results.

Preparation time
5 minutes

Cooking time
None

Servings
2 servings

Ingredients

- 1 cup strawberries
- 3/4 cup nonfat milk
- 4/5 cup diced pineapple
- 1 tsp. vanilla extract
- 2 tsp. honey
- 6 ice cubes (you can use a whole banana to thicken your mixture instead of ice)

Preparation:

Step 1: Blend the strawberries, milk, diced pineapple, vanilla extract, ice, and honey in a blender until smooth. You may need to scrape down the sides of the blender a couple of times to have a perfectly ground smoothie.

Step 2: Serve immediately.

Banana-coconut Smoothie

A morning protein smoothie is a great way to start the day. This shake will keep you full and give you energy until lunchtime. Just make sure not to add any extra sugar or sweeteners.

Preparation time
7 minutes

Cooking time
None

Servings
2 Servings

Ingredients

- 1/2 cup milk (almond, soy, etc.)
- 1 diced banana
- 3 tbsp. low-fat yogurt
- 1 diced green delicious apple
- 3 ice cubes

Preparation

Step 1: Blend all the ingredients in your blender.

Step 2: Serve immediately.

Mighty Smoothie

The mighty smoothie is full of antioxidants, which are necessary for a good flush of toxins out of your bloodstream. Include berries in most smoothies, and you will never regret your decision.

Preparation time
7 minutes

Cooking time
None

Servings
2 Servings

Ingredients

- 2 oranges (peel and pith removed and cut into chunks)
- 1 cup frozen blueberries
- 1 cup frozen raspberries

Preparation

Step 1: Combine all ingredients in a blender, and blend until smooth.

Step 2: Serve immediately.

Avocado Smoothie

As we all know, avocados include healthy fat that our body desperately needs to repair our tissues and also provide other health benefits. Avocados not only are used for guacamole, but in smoothies too. They are delicious and great to get your recommended vitamin intake for a great morning.

Preparation time
7 minutes

Cooking time
None

Servings
2 Servings

Ingredients

- 1 ripe avocado (halved and diced)
- 1 cup of nonfat milk
- 1/2 cup of nonfat yogurt
- 1 tsp. vanilla extract
- 3 tsp. honey
- 6 ice cubes

Preparation

Step 1: Combine the avocado, milk, yogurt, vanilla extract, ice cubes, and honey in a blender; blend until smooth.

Step 2: Serve immediately.

Detox Recipes

Detoxing the colon is fun and easy through juicing! Apples and lemons are an excellent choice for a detox recipe as they both are known to help cleanse the colon. You can also include beets, carrots, celery, ginger, and radishes. Almost any juice you make will help heal your body, so feel free to use whatever items you really enjoy.

The Green Cleanser

You should try to drink your vegetable juice at room temperature. This means you should take your vegetables out of the fridge and place them on the counter for a few hours before juicing. Ideally, and if you can, leave your vegetables out overnight to ensure they are at room temperature. In case you are new to juicing, begin with small doses. Start with vegetables that you ordinarily like, and slowly begin to introduce those that you enjoy less thoroughly. If you are juicing with a vegetable you aren't supposed to, your body will send you clear signals! Be sure to listen to your body, and you will enjoy your juicing experience.

Preparation time
7 minutes

Cooking time
None

Servings
2 Servings

Ingredients

- 1 large handful of fresh baby spinach
- 1 apple
- 3 carrots
- 1/2 cucumber

- 1/2 ginger
- 1 tbsp. flaxseed

Step 1: Wash your ingredients if necessary and blend them in your blender.

Step 2: Serve immediately.

The Mixer

People who want to juice but who have acid reflux, problems with candida like thrush, diabetes, or intestinal issues should avoid putting too much fruit into their recipes. Green items such as kale, parsley, chard, and broccoli will change the pH of the body to a healthier level, lowering your pH and blood sugar.

Preparation time
5 minutes

Cooking time
None

Servings
2 Servings

Ingredients

- 1 large handful of kale
- 1 apple
- 2 carrots
- 1 cucumber
- 1 tbsp. pumpkin seeds

Preparation

Step 1: Blend your ingredients and divide in two serving juice glasses.

Step 2: Serve immediately

Bright Skin

If you have an acne-prone skin, consider drinking freshly made carrot and spinach juice. Carrots contain high amounts of beta-carotene. Consumption of beta-carotene is absolutely critical if you want to clear up your skin. Spinach contains nutrients that make it a great blood cleanser and skin regenerator. Have a glass of carrot-spinach juice every day and see if it helps clear up your skin.

Preparation time
5 minutes

Cooking time
None

Servings
2 Servings

Ingredients

- 1 large handful spinach
- 1 cup cabbage
- 1 large tomato
- 1 tbsp. pumpkin seeds
- 1 carrot

Preparation

Step 1: Blend your ingredients and divide the mixture in two serving juice glasses.

Step 2: Serve immediately

Sweet Detox

Celery and cucumber are known to hold many nutrients, vitamins, and other benefits that are vital to good health.

Preparation time
4-6 minutes

Cooking time
None

Servings
2 Servings

Ingredients

- 3 apples
- 1 carrot
- 2 celery stalks
- 1/2 cucumber

Preparation

Step 1: Blend your ingredients and divide in two serving juice glasses.

Step 2: Serve immediately.

The Healer

If Alzheimer's disease runs in your family, you can use juice as a healthy way to slow the progress of the disease or even keep it away entirely. Recipes should include alfalfa, broccoli, cabbage (like the recipe below), kelp, onion, pumpkin (or seeds), or watercress to give you the best anti-Alzheimer's health boost you possibly can get in each drink. If you have an ulcer, try cabbage juice! It's been shown to help heal an ulcer while you're treating it with traditional medicine, to speed up your treatment. Many fruits and vegetables can help heal a variety of ailments, so do some research to find what can alleviate your predicament!

Preparation time
5 minutes

Cooking time
None

Servings
2 Servings

Ingredients

- 1 large handful spinach
- 1 cup cabbage
- 1 large tomato
- 1 tbsp. pumpkin seeds
- 1 carrot
- 1/2 tsp. lemon

Step 1: Blend your ingredients and divide the mixture in two serving juice glasses.

Step 2: Serve immediately.

Block my Hunger

Celery is a diuretic that helps the body shed water and diminish craving due to its high fiber content. It is also a great source of naturally occurring sodium, which can help the body maintain its careful balance while you are fasting.

Preparation time
5 minutes

Cooking time
None

Servings
2 Servings

Ingredients

- 3 stalks celery
- 2 cups spinach
- 2 cucumbers
- 1 green apple
- 1/2 jalapeño (optional)

Preparation

Step 1: Blend your ingredients and divide in two serving juice glasses.

Step 2: Serve immediately.

Weight-Loss Juicing Recipes

Use your juicing as part of a weight-loss plan to see big results. Fresh juice made from your fruits and veggies alone tends to be low in calories. It can be a helpful addition to your weight-loss plans. The fibrous nature of most veggies will help fill you up without adding in too many extra calories. When juicing for weight loss, it is important to eat the pulp, too. When using juicing as part of your weight-loss program, make sure you're doing it at a time that works best for you. Work it into your life as best you can, so if you can only do it every other day, it's better than nothing! Make sure to be tested regularly and stay under the care of a medical professional while attempting this as treatment.

Perfect Balance

Produce to use are apples, blueberries, garlic, kale, or kiwi, which all have nutrients that will reduce bad cholesterol in the blood. Adding blueberries in your juice will up your antioxidants and other vital nutrients. Make your own batch of juice geared to fit your own tastes.

Preparation time
5 minutes

Cooking time
None

Servings
2 Servings

Ingredients

- 2 apples
- 1 pear
- 1 beet
- 1 kiwi

- 1 cup blueberries
- 1 tsp. pumpkin seeds (optional)

Preparation

Step 1: Blend your ingredients and divide the mixture in two serving juice glasses.

Step 2: Serve immediately.

Green Monster

Lettuce juice is great for weight loss. The lettuce helps moderate the appetite. Some of the best, most nutritious lettuces to use are low-carb: romaine, spinach, and cabbage. Darker lettuces will have a strong taste and may need to be cut with other juices. Carrots are high in Vitamin A and beta-carotene. Add them to your green juices to boost an enjoyable taste to your juices.

Preparation time
4 minutes

Cooking time
None

Servings
2 Servings

Ingredients

- 1 apple
- 1 handful cabbage
- 3 carrots
- 1 cucumber
- 1 cup romaine lettuce
- Pumpkin seeds (optional)

Preparation

Step 1: Blend your ingredients and divide in two serving juice glasses.

Step 2: Serve immediately.

Spicy Kick

Maintaining blood sugar levels helps curb hunger, so including carrots in your juice creations helps keep you healthy and your hunger under control. Carrots do have more sugar in them than many other vegetables, but the fact that they don't cause a spike in blood glucose means you can overlook that and drink up!

Preparation time
5 minutes

Cooking time
None

Servings
2 Servings

Ingredients

- 1 cup of kale
- 1 apple
- 3 carrots
- 1 cucumber
- 1 inch piece of ginger
- 1 tsp. sunflower

Preparation

Step 1: Blend all of your ingredients and divide the mixture in two serving juice glasses.

Step 2: Serve immediately

Sweet and Bitter

When you are juicing, there are a few things that are important to remember to remove from the fruit you are using. The peel on oranges and grapefruit is bitter and will make your juice bitter as well. Additionally, remove any large seeds, such as those found in peaches or grapefruits, and stems included.

Preparation time
5 minutes

Cooking time
None

Servings
2 Servings

Ingredients

- 1 grapefruit
- 20 grapes
- 1 1/2 cup blueberries
- 5 strawberries
- 1 tsp. honey

Preparation

Step 1: Blend all of your ingredients and divide the mixture in two serving juice glasses.

Step 2: Serve immediately.

Rejuvenate Me

Cucumber included in juices has a very light and refreshing taste. Two of its benefits are skin rejuvenation and hair growth. Include it in most of your green recipes to get more health benefits.

Preparation time
5 minutes

Cooking time
None

Servings
2 Servings

Ingredients

- 1/2 cucumber
- 3 carrots
- 1 apple (with skin)
- 2 large handfuls of spinach
- 1/2 cup cabbage

Preparation

Step 1: Blend all of your ingredients and divide in two serving juice glasses.

Step 2: Serve immediately.

Fight That Cancer

Cantaloupe is one of the most nutritious fruits. Include it in your fruit recipes to reinforce your cancer-fighting cells and promote great health for the future.

Preparation time
4 minutes

Cooking time
None

Servings
2 Servings

Ingredients

- 1 cantaloupe
- 10 diced strawberries
- 1 cup blueberries
- 1 tsp. honey
- 1 tsp. sunflower

Preparation

Step 1: Wash your ingredients and blend them in your blender; divide in two serving juice glasses.

Step 2: Serve immediately.

Clear my Skin

This recipe not only helps you lose weight, but it also helps you treat acne and restore your skin to its normal state. Have this drink 3-5 times a week to see results.

Preparation time
5 minutes

Cooking time
None

Servings
2 Servings

Ingredients

- 1 watercress
- 1 apricot
- 1 cup of diced pumpkin
- 12 strawberries

Preparation

Step 1: Blend all of your ingredients and divide them in two serving juice glasses.

Step 2: Serve immediately.

Easy Digestion

This mixture not only helps you lose weight, but it also promotes great digestion. It is recommended to consume it first thing in the morning for the best results.

Preparation time
5 minutes

Cooking time
None

Servings
2 Servings

Ingredients

- 2 apples
- 3 carrots
- 4 celery stalks

Preparation

Step 1: Blend all of your ingredients and divide them in two serving juice glasses.

Step 2: Serve immediately.

Flush It Out

Beets regenerate red blood cells and are fantastic for flushing toxins, but should be used in the company of other fruits or vegetables to make up the majority of the drink.

Preparation time
5 minutes

Cooking time
None

Servings
2 Servings

Ingredients

- 1/2 cucumber
- 1 diced beet
- 1 tsp. pumpkin seeds
- 1 tsp. honey (optional)

Preparation

Step 1: Blend all of your ingredients and divide them in two serving juice glasses.

Step 2: Serve immediately

Soups Recipes

Onion Soup

Onion soup is a light meal that is mostly consumed at night. It is usually served when guests begin to feel fatigued. The real recipe is prepared with water instead of beef stock.

Preparation time
20 minutes

Cooking time
1 hour

Servings
6 Servings

Ingredients

- 2 oz. butter
- 1 1/2 lbs. onion, thinly sliced
- 10 oz. (2 cans) beef stock
- 1/2 tsp. salt
- French bread or hard toast
- 1 cup of grated Swiss or Gruyere cheese
- 1 tsp. cognac or brandy

Preparation

Step 1: Slice the onions thinly.

Step 2: Melt the butter in a skillet and cook the onions for 15 minutes until lightly browned over medium heat.

Step 3: Stir the flour and gently blend it with the thinly sliced onions.

Step 4: Add the beef stock and the cognac or brandy. Boil the mixture, reducing the heat to low. Cover and let it simmer for twenty to thirty minutes.

Step 5: Toast the bread at 325°F or 165°F.

Step6: Serve the soup into bowls, float the bread, and add the cheese. If the bowls are oven-proof, place them under the broiler to brown the cheese.

Cherry Soup

This is a traditional soup that is mostly served in the winter. To make the soup more flavorful, several suggest adding lemon juice, red wine, or cinnamon.

Preparation time
7 minutes

Cooking time
None

Servings
2 Servings

Ingredients

- 2 tsp. cherry brandy
- 1 3/4 lb. black cherries
- 1 tsp. cornstarch or corn flour
- 3 tsp. sugar (consider using a sweetener instead)
- Water
- 6 slices of bread

Preparation

Step 1: Clean and drain the cherries. Remove the stems.

Step 2: Place cherries in a saucepan with sugar and cherry brandy. Bring to a boil over medium heat and cook for 15 minutes.

Step 3: Melt 1 1/2 tablespoons of butter in a skillet. Add bread slices and saute until browned on both sides. Drain on paper towel. Add more butter if needed to brown all the slices.

Step 4: In a bowl, blend 1 tsp. of corn flour and 1 tbsp. of water.

Step 5: Remove the cherries from the pan, using a spoon. Add to the pan the mixture of corn flour and water. Stir well over low heat for a few minutes.

Step 6: Return the cherries to the pan for a few seconds.

Step7: Put the bread slices in a bowl. Pour the soup over the bread.

Lobster Soup

This dish is mouthwatering and delicious. It can be consumed with red wine or water if you are at work. Vegetarians are welcome to enjoy this meal as well!

Preparation time
20 minutes

Cooking time
60 minutes

Servings
4 Servings

Ingredients

- 4 oz. carrots
- Salt
- 2 cooked lobsters of 1 lb. each
- 2 oz. celery stalks
- 2 pints fish stock
- 4 oz. flour
- 3 cloves garlic
- 1 oz. tomato purée
- 13 fl. oz. white wine
- cayenne pepper
- crème fraîche or whipping cream
- 4 oz. onions
- 3 fl. oz. brandy
- 3 fl. oz. olive oil
- Lentils
- Turkey bacon

Preparation

Step 1: Remove the lobster meat from the shells. Dice one lobster tail and refrigerate until ready to serve. Use the remaining lobster meat in another recipe or freeze for later use. Chop the lobster shells into small pieces.

Step 2: Peel and slice the onion, and chop the celery and carrots. Peel and crush the garlic.

Step 3: Place the lentils, onions, carrots, bacon, and herbs in a large pan. Cover with cold water, add salt, and bring to a boil. When the water is boiling, turn the heat down and cook gently for 40 minutes.

Step 4: Heat the olive oil in a large pan, and saute the onions, celery, carrots, and garlic until tender. Add the chopped lobster shells and cook for 8 minutes, stirring frequently. Add the tomato purée and cook for a further 5 minutes, stirring constantly. Add the flour to the pan and cook for an additional 3 minutes. Pour in the brandy, white wine, and fish stock and season with salt and cayenne pepper. Bring to a boil and skim frequently to remove any impurities. Lower the heat and cook gently for 45 minutes.

Step 5: Puree the mixture in a food processor. Pass it through a fine sieve.

Step6: Put the soup back on the heat and cook until it begins to bubble. Adjust seasoning if required.

Step7: Divide the soup among six bowls. Top with a dollop of crème fraîche and the diced lobster-tail meat.

Step8: Serve with red or white wine to increase the tastiness of the dish

Watercress Soup

Watercress soup is a simple recipe that is made with leeks and potatoes. It is really healthy and has a lot vitamins and minerals.

Preparation time
15 minutes

Cooking time
45 minutes

Servings
6 Servings

Ingredients

- 1/4 lb. watercress
- 5 tbsp. whipping cream
- 1 lb. sliced leeks
- 1 lb. diced potatoes
- 2 quarts water
- Salt

Preparation

Step 1: Simmer the leeks and potatoes with a pinch of salt in water for 40 minutes.

Step 2: Add the watercress and simmer for 5 minutes.

Step 3: Off the heat, mash the vegetables with a fork. Add salt if needed.

Step 4: Stir in the whipping cream just before serving.

Suggestion

Use a few watercress leaves to decorate. Boil them for 30 seconds in water, drain, and decorate the plates.

La Soupe Au Potiron (Pumpkin Soup)

Nothing else matters when you are in the presence of a tasty soup like La Soupe au Potiron or pumpkin soup. This soup is a delicacy and is mostly consumed in the fall, but it is really not a crime to enjoy it during the winter or spring. It is very healthy and adds a lot of vitamins to your diet during your process of weight loss. It is easy to cook and inexpensive, especially when you get the ingredients from your local farmers' market. Have fun with it and enjoy the benefits of French cuisine and your LDL reduction!

Preparation time
15 minutes

Cooking time
45 minutes

Servings
6 Servings

Ingredients

- 2 1/2 lbs. pumpkin
- 2 pints vegetable stock
- Salt
- Ground pepper
- 2 onions
- 6 sprigs chervil
- 7 fl. oz. heavy cream or crème fraîche
- 3 pinches ground coriander
- 1 pinch ground nutmeg
- 3 oz. butter

Preparation

Step 1: Cut up the pumpkin and remove all the seeds and pulp. Cut off the skin and then cut the flesh into small chunks. Take about 3 1/2 oz. of the pumpkin flesh, dice, and place aside. Peel and finely dice the onions. Make sure you save a couple of pieces for decoration. About 24 pieces would be enough for six servings.

Step 2: Melt half the butter in a pot and fry the onions for 5 minutes. Next, add the pumpkin pieces and fry on a low heat for 5 minutes, stirring constantly. Sprinkle on the nutmeg, coriander, salt, and pepper.

Step 3: Cook gently for 5 minutes, stirring all the time to ensure that the soup does not stick to the pan. Pour on the stock and cook on a low heat for a further 20 minutes until the pumpkin is soft.

Step 4: Pour the soup into a mixing bowl and mix with an electric mixer, adding the crème fraîche or heavy cream until you achieve a smooth, creamy consistency; then place it aside.

Step 5: Brown the diced pumpkin saved earlier in a pan with butter, then season with a little salt and pepper to taste.

Step6: Share the soup among six bowls and the browned diced pumpkin. Decorate with a sprig of chervil for each plate and some ground pepper, and serve straightaway. In case your dinner is delayed, just before serving, gently reheat the soup without boiling.

La Soupe Aux Choux (Cabbage Soup)

Soupe aux choux, also referred as cabbage soup, is the ultimate weight-loss in nutrition! It is rich in vegetables and at the same time provides essential proteins and vitamins that your body needs for optimal health. Soupe aux choux is vegetarian-friendly and can be consumed daily.

Preparation time
15 minutes

Cooking time
45 minutes

Servings
6 Servings

Ingredients

- 6 onions
- 2 peeled tomatoes
- 1 cabbage
- 2 green peppers
- 2 celery sticks
- 500ml of vegetable broth
- 2 bay leaves
- 1 cup cooked kidney beans
- 1 tsp. curry powder
- 6 sprigs cilantro
- Salt
- Pepper

Preparation

Step 1: Cut the vegetables, including the cabbage, into small pieces and bring to a boil, adding the vegetable broth, salt, pepper, curry powder, and bay leaves.

Step 2: Cook the mixture for 10 minutes or until the vegetables are tender.

Step 3: Add the cooked kidney beans.

Step 4: Serve and decorate with one piece of cilantro for each bowl.

Note: You also can add tofu in the dishes instead of kidney beans.

Main Course

Beef Liver (Foie de Génisse) Purses

As you might be aware, beef liver is rich in vitamins and protein essential for a healthy body. Beef liver contains about 130 calories, with about 3.6g of fat, which should be enough for your daily intake. One slice of liver contains more than 430% of Vitamin A, 137% percent of Vitamin B12, 59.6% of niacin, 48.3% of Vitamin B5, 34.6% of Vitamin B6, nearly 800% of B12, 338mg of phosphorus, and nearly 25% of iron. Iron is really essential in the creation of red blood cells and allows oxygen to be transported into your body as well. All these vitamins and minerals can be found in this dish. Weight loss should not be your only concern; health and good skin texture have to follow. Luckily, beef liver purses are not only nutritional, but it is inexpensive as well! In case you are a vegetarian or a vegan, use cooked beans instead of liver. You can consume it as many times as you want and lose the excess weight. Have fun with this dish and enjoy the recipe with friends and family.

Preparation time
20 minutes

Cooking time
1 hour

Servings
6 Servings

Ingredients

- 1/2 beef liver
- 4 grated carrots
- 2 tbsp. olive oil
- 6 crepes
- 3 leeks
- 1 oz. butter

- 1 big shallot
- Salt
- Pepper

Preparation

Step 1: Wash the liver, thinly slice it, and set it aside.

Step 2: Wash the leeks. Thinly slice two of them. Cut the third one into wide slices lengthwise.

Step 3: In a frying pan, add one teaspoon of butter and one tablespoon of olive oil, then throw in the sliced liver, salt, and pepper and cook for 5 minutes.

Step 4: At the end of the 5 minutes, add the carrots and the thinly sliced leeks, and cook for ten minutes or until the liver has no traces of blood. Stir constantly!

Step 5: Peel and slice the shallot and throw it in the liver and cook for another two minutes on low heat.

Step6: Reheat the crepes in a bit of butter and spread them on the work surface. Fill them with the cooked liver mixture, close the crepes to make a purse shape, and tie it up with one of the leek strips.

Step7: Serve immediately!

Turkey Bacon with Parsley

The cost of this dish is minimal. It is rich in vitamins. You could remove the turkey bacon in case you are a vegetarian and replace it with tofu or beans (kidney beans) instead. To make the meal a bit heavy, consume it with pita bread or cooked sweet potatoes. Serve it for dinner and have fun with your family!

Preparation time
180 minutes

Cooking time
3 hour

Servings
2 Servings

Ingredients

- 2 carrots
- 3 tbsp. white wine vinegar
- freshly ground pepper
- 1 bunch flat parsley
- 1 bouquet garni (bunch of thyme and bay leaf)
- 4 slice of low-fat turkey bacon
- 1 tsp. black peppercorns
- 3 cloves
- Salt
- 4 cloves garlic
- 1 tbsp. rose pepper
- 1 pint white wine
- 1 shallot

Preparation

Step 1: Desalinate the turkey bacon for twenty-four hours by placing it in cold water and changing the water regularly.

Step 2: The following day, peel and slice the carrots. Peel the onion and stud it with the cloves. Peel and quarter the shallot. Peel the clove of garlic. Wash and dry the parsley and drain the turkey bacon. Save one-third of the parsley and garlic for further use.

Step 3: In a large pot, place the onion, shallot, garlic (peeled), three sprigs of parsley, the bouquet garni, the black peppercorns, and the turkey bacon. Pour on the white wine and add enough water to just cover all the ingredients. Gently bring to boil on low heat, skimming regularly. Cover and leave to simmer over low heat for two hours.

Step 4: Peel the carrots and cut them into chunks, then add them to the pot and cook for another hour. Add the vinegar to the stock and check the seasoning, then leave it to cool.

Step 5: Remove the stalks from the remaining parsley and chop finely. Peel and finely chop the remaining garlic. Add the parsley and garlic to the stock and mix well.

Step6: Sprinkle on the rose pepper, cover with the mixture, and refrigerate for twenty-four hours.

Step7: Serve immediately with bread or warm potatoes.

Sarladaise Salad

Sarladaise salad is prepared with various vegetables and beans. The original dish is cooked with expensive items, but I have switched it with affordable groceries so everyone can enjoy! Enjoy this meal as many times as you want daily or weekly! It is low in LDL fat and high in vitamins and minerals. Roquefort cheese can be found at Whole Foods Markets locations.

Preparation time
20 minutes

Cooking time
20 minutes

Servings
6 Servings

Ingredients

- 5 oz. chopped low-fat turkey bacon
- 12 slices smoked turkey meat (boneless)
- 1 romaine lettuce (curly)
- 5 oz. string green beans
- 5 oz. Roquefort cheese
- 5 oz. mushrooms
- Pepper
- Salt
- 1 small bunch chives
- 4 potatoes
- 4 tbsp. olive oil
- 1 tbsp. pine nuts

Preparation

Step 1: Peel the potatoes and slice them thinly. Top and tail the green beans and remove any strings. Clean the mushrooms. Crumble the Roquefort. Wash, dry, and chop the chives.

Step 2: Cook the beans for 15 minutes in boiling salted water. Then remove it and transfer it immediately into ice water to avoid losing the greenness of the vegetable.

Step 3: Heat the oil in a nonstick pan and fry the potato slices in it.

Step 4: When they start to brown, add the bacon and the mushrooms. Stir until cooked and then drain on kitchen paper.

Step 5: Wash and dry the lettuce.

Step6: In a large bowl, mix the lettuce, potatoes, bacon, mushrooms, green beans, Roquefort, and pine nuts. Add salt and pepper and serve.

Lentil Savories with Mushrooms

This recipe is easy to make, and it is inexpensive in terms of your budget. Vegetarians are welcome to enjoy this meal!

Preparation time
20 minutes

Cooking time
60 minutes

Servings
4 Servings

Ingredients

- 2 cups mushrooms
- 8 peppercorns
- 12 oz. green lentils
- 2 cloves garlic
- 2 small bouquet garni (bunch of thyme and bay leaves)
- 2 carrots
- 2 cloves
- 4 sprigs parsley
- ground pepper
- 2 onions

Preparation

Step 1: Twenty minutes prior to starting the recipe, cook the mushrooms for 10 minutes and cool it in icy water.

Step 2: Meanwhile, peel and slice the carrots. Peel the onions and pierce them with the cloves.

Step 3: Place the lentils, onions, carrots, and herbs in a large pan. Cover with cold water, add salt, and bring to a boil. When the water is boiling, turn the heat down and cook gently for 40 minutes.

Step 4: When the lentils are cooked, drain them and remove the onions and herbs. Put the lentils aside and keep warm.

Step 5: Place the lentils in one large pot, with a thick base. Douse them in the cooking juices from the mushrooms, which should be thickened, add pepper, and cook with the lid on for 20 minutes.

Step6: Place in a dish and serve.

Eggs Stuffed with Tuna

I particularly love this recipe because it is quick to prepare and inexpensive. The richness of the eggs gives it a great taste. It is suitable for every season and very healthy for an individual on a diet. Take out the egg yolk if you are on a restricted diet.

Preparation time
15 minutes

Cooking time
10 minutes

Servings
4 Servings

Ingredients

- 1 can tuna
- 4 stalks chives
- Pepper
- 4 eggs
- 1 sprig coriander
- 2 tbsp. lemon dressing
- Salt

Preparation

Step 1: Submerge the eggs in boiling salt water and cook for 10 minutes.

Step 2: Meanwhile, drain and crumble the tuna. Add the lemon dressing, season, and mix.

Step 3: Remove the leaves from the coriander and wash and dry them. Wash, dry, and chop the chives.

Step 4: Drain the eggs and place in cold water. Remove the shells and cut them in two. Take out the yolks and crumble them into the tuna mixture. Mix briskly.

Step 5: Place the egg whites in a dish and stuff the hollow left by the yolk with a little of the tuna mixture. Sprinkle on the chopped chives and decorate with a few coriander leaves.

Step 6: Serve.

Hot and Cold Crab

This dish is a bit expensive. In order to have the perfect taste and freshness of the food, it has to be made with fresh crabs. The difficulty in cooking this recipe is moderate. The recipe is very healthy if done without any high-fat oil content. The dish is mostly served during the summer, but I enjoy it all year long!

Preparation time
25 minutes

Cooking time
30 minutes

Servings
4 Servings

Ingredients

- 4 pinches pre-cooked crab claws
- 6 potatoes
- Pepper
- Sea salt
- 1 tin crab meat
- 3 sprigs flat-leaf parsley
- 2 sprigs dill
- 3 tbsp. olive oil

Preparation

Step 1: Place the potatoes in a pan of cold salty water. Bring to a boil and cook for 30 minutes.

Step 2: Meanwhile, break and carefully remove the shell of the crab claws. Draw out the flesh from the claws.

Step 3 Crumble the tinned crab meat into a bowl. Wash, dry, and chop the herbs, having first removed any stalks. Mix with the olive oil.

Step 4: Drain the potatoes. Peel them and roughly mash them with a fork. Place them in a pan, and add half of the herb-infused olive oil, some sea salt, and some pepper.

Step 5: Take four ramekins and make a layer of the potato mixture in each. Add the crab pieces and press down hard. Turn each mold out onto a plate and cover with the crumbled crab meat. Drizzle some herb oil around each and serve immediately.

Leeks with Vinaigrette

This recipe is budget-friendly and has a lot of flavor, which melts completely in the mouth after each bite. It is very easy to cook and is mostly served in the winter. If you are looking for a great vegetarian dish, this will be your best choice.

Preparation time
20 minutes

Cooking time
20 minutes

Servings
6 Servings

Ingredients

- Pepper
- Garlic
- 1 small bunch chives
- 12 leeks
- 2 onions
- 1 tbsp. xérès (or sherry) vinegar (red wine vinegar will also work)
- 3 tbsp. hazelnut oil
- Salt

Preparation

Step 1: Clean the leeks. Cut off the dark green tops of the leeks and tie the leeks into two bundles of six each. Prepare a large pan of salted water and bring to a boil. Immerse the leek bundles in the water and cook for 20 minutes.

Step 2: Drain the leeks and undo the bundles. Place the leeks in a dish and allow them to cool.

Step 3: Meanwhile, peel and dice the onions and garlic. Wash, dry, and chop the chives.

Step 4: Heat a tablespoon of oil in a frying pan and swiftly fry the chopped onion, garlic, and chives for 5 minutes, stirring frequently. Take off the heat and leave to cool.

Step 5: Mix the garlic, onion, and chives with the hazelnut oil and the xérès vinegar.

Step 6: Add salt and pepper.

Step 7: Pour the vinaigrette over the leeks and serve either hot or cold.

Moules Mariniere (Mussels in wine sauce)v

Moules is French for mussels. This is a delicate dish. It can be paired with sauteed French green beans or sauteed onions. Mussels need to be steamed in only a tiny amount of liquid. When they open during cooking, they release their own liquid, which adds a lot of liquid to the base sauce. If there is too much liquid in the sauce before adding the mussels, the liquid from the mussels will dilute the sauce. Be careful when seasoning the sauce as the liquid from the mussels tends to be quite salty and will season the sauce on its own. Red or white wine is recommended for a great taste!

Preparation time
20 minutes

Cooking time
20 minutes

Servings
6 Servings

Ingredients

- 2 lb. mussels
- 1/3 cup shallots
- 2 cloves garlic
- 1/4 cup Italian flat-leaf parsley
- 1/4 cup unsalted butter
- 1/2 cup dry white wine
- Salt (to taste)
- Freshly ground black pepper (to taste)

Preparation

Step 1: To start your mise en place, first mince the shallots and garlic. Roughly chop the parsley and set it aside, along with the butter and white wine.

Step 2: Prepare the mussels by scrubbing them clean and removing any beards. Place into a bowl and cover with a damp cloth. Store the mussels in the refrigerator while you make the sauce.

Step 3: To make the sauce, heat a large, wide pan (with a lid) over medium heat. Add the butter. Once melted, add the shallots. Sweat (saute in a covered vessel until natural juices are exuded) for about 3 minutes or until translucent, but not browned. Next, add the garlic and cook for about 30 seconds. Add the white wine, turn up the heat to medium-high, and let the mixture reduce for a few minutes. Once the sauce has reduced and almost all of the liquid has evaporated, add a pinch of salt and pepper.

Step 4: Now add the mussels. Cover immediately with a lid and turn the heat down to medium. Let it cook for 6-8 minutes or until the mussels open. Once done, sprinkle the chopped parsley over the top.

Step 5: To serve, pour the mussels into a large bowl, with soup plates for diner. Serve with fresh bread to soak up all of the delicious sauce.

Olive Tapenade

This recipe is mainly made with olives, olive oil, garlic, and pepper, which is where it derives its name.

Preparation time
10 minutes

Cooking time
None

Servings
6 Servings

Ingredients

- 1 1/2 cup black olives
- Fresh black pepper
- 2 garlic gloves
- 2 1/2 oz. anchovy fillets (also great with salmon fillet)
- 1/2 cup capers
- 1/2 cup olive oil

Preparation

Step 1: Drain capers. Peel garlic. Pit olives.

Step 2: Put olives, anchovy fillets, garlic cloves, and capers in a food processor or mortar. Mix until the mixture is a paste.

Step 3: Slowly add the olive oil and black pepper. Continue to mix until the paste is creamy.

Step 4: Cover with a film. Refrigerate.

Serving: Tapenade can be stored in a refrigerator for only two weeks. Tapenade is excellent on bread and toast, but also with potatoes; sweet potatoes are best for dieters.

Verrines Bayadère

This dish is a combination of all vegetables. It could be a little expensive to prepare, but it is worth it. You can make it for a romantic dinner. This recipe will be perfect for vegetarians!

Preparation time
20 minutes

Cooking time
30 minutes

Servings
6 Servings

Ingredients

- 1 lb. salmon fillet, skinned and boned (if you do not consume seafood, replace it with tomatoes instead)
- 1 bunch green asparagus
- 3/4 fromage frais
- 1 bunch chervil
- 1 bunch fennel
- 2 tsp. of single cream (could be replaced by plain yogurt)
- 5 tsp. olive oil
- 2 tsp. lemon juice
- 1 small pot lump-fish eggs (leave it out if you are allergic or have some concerns)
- Salt
- Pepper

Preparation

Step 1: Peel the asparagus. Cut off the tips and put them aside. Cut the stalks into chunks, and immerse them in boiling water. Cook them for 20 minutes. Drain them and leave them to cool.

Step 2: Wash, dry, and pluck the chervil.

Step 3: Place the asparagus pieces in an electric mixer. Add 4 tsp. of olive oil and the chervil, and season with salt and pepper. Pulse until it is thoroughly minced and put it aside.

Step 4: Wash, dry, and plunk the fennel. Place the fromage frais in a mixer and add single cream and fennel. Season the mixture with salt and pepper, and mix until the mixture is of an even texture. Finally place it in the fridge.

Step 5: Chop the salmon into small pieces and then coarsely mince with a knife. Place it in a mixing bowl and add the lemon juice and the olive oil to it. Season with salt and pepper, mix well, and refrigerate.

Step6: Steam the asparagus tips for 10 minutes and let them cool. Next, cut them in two lengthwise.

Step 7: Arrange the mixture in consecutive layers in glasses. Decorate with lump-fish eggs, asparagus tips, and sprigs of fennel.

Useful Tips: Serve chilled! For a better celebratory meal, decorate with caviar instead of lump-fish eggs.

Crunchy Green Tomato, Cucumber and Whole-Wheat Bread

The name explains it. It is a mixture of vegetables, and bread for decoration at the end of the recipe.

Preparation time
20 minutes

Cooking time
1 hour 10 minutes

Servings
6 Servings

Ingredients

- 1 1/2 stick butter
- 3 1/2 oz. shelled peas (should be uncooked)
- 1 sprig rosemary
- 2 tbsp. vinegar
- 6 tsp. olive oil
- 6 green tomatoes
- 6 thinly sliced pieces whole-wheat bread
- Salt
- Ground pepper
- 1 cucumber
- 3 tsp. honey
- Sesame seeds

Preparation

Step 1: Boil water and season it with salt and a sprig of rosemary in a skillet. Add the peas and cook until they are slightly tender, and then refresh them in cold water. Place the mixture aside.

Step 2: Wash and dry the tomatoes and cut them into quarters. Remove the seeds and dice them finely. Place them in a mixing bowl, and season with salt and pepper. Pour vinegar and olive oil into the mixture. Mix, and place it aside.

Step 3: Peel the cucumber, cut it in two lengthwise removing the seeds, and then dice finely. Add the cucumber, along with the peas, to the diced tomatoes. Mix well and season the mixture, then cover and chill in the fridge for an hour.

Step 4: Preheat the oven to 390ºF.

Step 5: Thinly slice the bread and glace it with melted butter and very lightly with honey using a pastry brush. Sprinkle the thinly sliced bread with sesame seeds. Place it in the oven for three minutes; keep a close eye on it, and as soon as it becomes hard enough as toasted bread, remove it.

Step6: Put the mixture on a plate and top it off with the baked bread; place the sliced cucumber on the top.

Calamari Ceviche

Calamari ceviche is among the Mediterranean recipes. It is healthy and tasty for someone on a diet. This type of dish is expensive to prepare, and it is \a once in-a-while kind of dish. It is easy to make and is mostly consumed in the summer. A clever tip is to cook the dish with sea bass, monkfish, or king prawns. White champagne or red or white wine is recommended. The higher you go for the price of your drink, the better your taste of the calamari will be! Again, visit your local farmers market for cheaper and more affordable dishes.

Preparation time
20 minutes

Cooking time
None

Servings
6 Servings

Ingredients

- 3 calamari
- 6 limes
- 1 bunch coriander
- 2 sticks citronella or 2 garlic cloves
- 1 red pepper
- 1 small red chili pepper
- Salt

Preparation

Step 1: Ask the fishmonger to clean and prepare the calamari.

Step 2: Wash the limes. Remove the zest with a potato peeler and press the juice.

Step 3: Finely dice the calamari and place them in a mixing bowl.

Step 4: Peel and finely chop the citronella or garlic. Wash and seed the pepper and finely dice it. Wash, dry, and pluck the coriander. Wash the chili, remove the seeds, and chop it finely.

Step 5: Add the zest, citronella, coriander, pepper, and chili to the calamari. Pour on the lime juice, season with salt, and mix well. Cover with a cling film and place in the fridge for at least 2 hours.

Step6: Serve the dish in six separate small bowls, along with tacos.

Onions and Leek Gratin

Onions and leek gratin is a very tasty dish made with Gruyere and bread. It is heavy and dinner-appropriate. Your family will enjoy this dish. It is full of vegetables, just like other dishes, and very nutritious. Enjoy it two or three times per week, and you will think twice before embracing your old habits again!

Preparation time
15 minutes

Cooking time
40 minutes

Servings
6 Servings

Ingredients

- 1 loaf French bread (can be found in Whole Foods stores)
- 1 stick salted butter or 4 tbsp. olive oil
- 1 tbsp. flour
- Salt
- 5 oz. grated Gruyere cheese
- 2 pints chicken stock
- 10 1/2 onions
- 3 leeks
- Pepper
- 6 oven-proof dishes

Preparation

Step 1: Peel and finely dice the onions. Wash and slice the leeks. Pour the chicken stock in a saucepan and warm it without boiling.

Step 2: Melt the butter in a cooking pot, and when it begins to froth, add the onions and leeks. Sweat (saute in a covered vessel until natural juices are exuded) the vegetables on high heat, for about 5 minutes, stirring constantly. Sprinkle them with flour, stir, and then add the stock. Season with salt and pepper and then lower the heat. Cover and cook gently for 30 minutes. Meanwhile, cut the French bread into slices and toast them. Preheat the grill.

Step 3: Distribute the soup among six oven-proof dishes. Place a few slices of bread on top and sprinkle with the grated cheese. Grill for about 5 minutes, with the oven door half open.

Step 4: Serve immediately!

Pasta and Sardine Salad

This is basically a pasta salad dish. It is considered an appetizer and can be very light since it is served in a small portion.

Preparation time
15 minutes

Cooking time
10 minutes

Servings
6 Servings

Ingredients

- 14 oz. small-sized pasta
- 1 fennel bulb
- 3 spring onions
- 1 tsp. capers
- 1 bunch basil
- Olive oil
- 2 tins sardines in olive oil
- Salt
- Pepper

Preparation

Step 1: Cook the pasta in boiling water seasoned with salt and a little olive oil. Cook it according to time indicated on the package.

Step 2: Drain and pour pasta into a mixing bowl.

Step 3: Drain the sardine fillets.

Step 4: Cut the base of the fennel, remove any damaged leaves, and slice it finely.

Step 5: Peel and finely dice the onions. Wash, dry, and pluck the basil.

Step6: Place half of the basil in a mortar and pestle. Add the capers and crush them, adding the olive oil until you get a thick sauce; season with salt and pepper.

Step7: Add the sardines, fennel, onions, and the sauce to the mixing bowl and mix well.

Step 8: Share the salad among the plates and decorate with basil leaves. Serve immediately.

Useful time: You can also marinate fresh sardine fillets in lemon juice and olive oil. You can share the sardine salad among the plates placing the marinated sauce on the top.

Prawn Salad

This dish is basically shrimp, vegetables, and fruits. To improve the flavor of this dish, I recommend you serve it with a glass of red wine! It helps you lose weight since it is only served in a small portion.

Preparation time
15 minutes

Cooking time
None

Servings
6 Servings

Ingredients

- 24 king prawns (shrimp)
- 1/2 cucumber
- 2 bananas
- 1 pink grapefruit
- 1 purple onion
- 1 handful fresh baby spinach
- 2 sprigs fennel
- Salt
- Pepper
- 1 handful of baby beetroot
- 1/2 lemon
- 5 tbsp. olive oil

Preparation

Step 1: Peel and skin the grapefruit. Detach the segments by sliding the blade of a serrated knife between the fine membranes to separate them. Cut the segments into small pieces.

Step 2: Wash the cucumber and then cut into very thin strips using a potato peeler. Peel and finely slice the onion. Wash and drain the beetroot and spinach leaves.

Step 3: Wash and dry the fennel and remove the stalks.

Step 4: Shell the prawns. Peel the banana and cut it into thin round pieces.

Step 5: Press the lemon juice, mix it with the olive oil, and season with salt and pepper.

Step6: Combine all the ingredients you have prepared in a mixing bowl. Pour on the freshly squeezed lemon sauce you have prepared and stir. Check the seasoning and serve chilled.

Step7: Serve the dish cold on small plates.

Winter Vegetables Casserole

This is a fruit and vegetable casserole. It is packed with vitamins and all the nutrients that your body might be craving. For this specific meal, you can add whatever spices or herbs you fancy to your casserole. Make sure that you add them at the end of the cooking process so that they keep their flavor. Red or white wine is recommended for this meal. This casserole is delicious and diet-friendly. As always, visit your local farmers market to make your meals inexpensively.

Preparation time
30 minutes

Cooking time
45 minutes

Servings
6 Servings

Ingredients

- 3 apples
- 3 pears
- 1/4 white cabbage
- 3 small leeks
- 3 chicory
- 1/4 pumpkin
- 2 red onions
- 1/2 stick salted butter
- 1 tbsp. oil
- 1 bouquet garni (bunch of thyme and bay leaves)
- Salt
- 1 tsp. peppercorns

Preparation

Step 1: Wash the pears and the apples. Cut them in two and remove the cores with a small pointed knife. Peel the pumpkin and cut it into slices. Cut the chicory in two. Peel the leeks and cut them in two. Separate the cabbage leaves and wash them. Peel and finely dice the onions.

Step 2: Gently heat the butter and the oil in a large pot. Add the apples, leeks, chicory, cabbage leaves, and onions. Fry for two minutes and then pour in the stock, add the bouquet garni and the peppercorns.

Step 3: Cover the pot and cook for 20 minutes over low heat. Add the pears and the pumpkin slices, and salt lightly. Cook for another 20 minutes, keeping the pot at a low heat with the lid on.

Step 4: Share the vegetables and fruit either among the plates or in mini-casserole dishes. Pour a little of the cooking juice on the dishes.

Step 5: Serve right away.

Ratatouille

Ratatouille is a combination of eggplant, zucchini, tomatoes, and onions. It is a very healthy dish and great for weight loss.

Preparation time
30 minutes

Cooking time
45 minutes

Servings
6 Servings

Ingredients

- 1 lb. eggplant
- 1 lb. zucchini
- 4 tbsp. olive oil
- 1/2 lb. yellow onions
- 2 garlic cloves
- 1 lb. tomatoes, firm and ripe
- 3 tbsp. parsley
- Salt and pepper

Preparation

Step 1: Peel and cut the eggplant into three-inch long slices. Cut the zucchini into slices, but don't peel. Place those vegetables in a bowl, cover with water, and let rest for thirty minutes. Drain.

Step 2: Sauté the eggplant and zucchini with olive oil in a skillet, one minute on each side. Set aside.

Step 3: Cook the onions with olive oil in the same skillet for ten minutes over moderate heat. Stir in the garlic and add salt and pepper.

Step 4: Peel the tomatoes and boil for thirty seconds. Cut into slices. Lay them over the onions in the skillet. Cover and cook over low heat for 5 minutes. Uncover. Pour the juice from the skillet over the tomatoes. Raise heat and boil for several minutes until juice has almost entirely evaporated.

Step 5: Put one-third of the tomato mixture in the bottom of a casserole. Sprinkle 1 tsp. of parsley. Then put half of the eggplant and zucchini in a casserole. Continue doing the same for the second and third layers of tomatoes. Sprinkle with 1 tbsp. of parsley. Put in the remaining eggplant and zucchini, then the tomatoes, and sprinkle with tbsp. of parsley.

Step 6: Cover and simmer over low heat for 10 minutes. Uncover; pour the juice over the vegetables. Add salt and pepper if needed. Raise heat to moderate and cook uncovered for 15 minutes. Pour the juice during the process several times over the vegetables.

Useful Tips: This dish can be served hot or cold.

Lamb Navarin

Lamb Navarin is a traditional stew with spring vegetables such as green peas and carrots. It may be called *navarin* because of the turnips in the recipe; *navet* in French means turnip.

Preparation time
20 minutes

Cooking time
1 hour 30 minutes

Servings
6 Servings

Ingredients

- 3 to 4 lb. of lamb (shoulder, neck, and breast)
- 2 tbsp. flour
- 3 cups lamb or beef stock
- 4 tomatoes, ripe, peeled, seeded, and chopped
- 5 carrots, peeled
- 5 turnips, peeled
- 12 spring onions
- 1 lb. green peas or snow peas
- 2 garlic gloves, mashed
- Herbs: 1 bay leaf, 1/4 tsp. thyme
- Salt and pepper
- Olive oil

Preparation

Step 1: Cut the lamb into 2" pieces.

Step 2: In a large saucepan or casserole, heat 1 tbsp. of oil. Brown over medium heat a few pieces of lamb at a time and saute until brown on all sides.

Step 3: Put all pieces of meat in the casserole, add garlic gloves, and cook over high heat for 1 minute.

Step 4: Remove one-half of the fat. Toss the meat with flour, salt, and pepper. Cook over high heat for 2minutes.

Step 5: Warm the stock in a different saucepan. Add to the meat. Boil. Stir. Add the tomatoes and herbs. Boil and simmer for 30 minutes over medium to low heat.

Step 6: Add the carrots, onions, and turnips. Simmer for 30 minutes again over medium to low heat.

Step 7: Cook the peas in a saucepan with salted water for 5 minutes. Add to the lamb just 5 minutes before serving. Remove the herbs.

Oxtail in Red Wine

This is an oxtail recipe. Make sure you remove all the fat from the meat before cooking it. If you are a vegetarian, you can replace it with mushrooms. This dish tastes even better if you prepare it a day before and reheat it an hour before serving. A red wine is recommended for this particular dish. It can be consumed in all four seasons of the year. It is moderately expensive to cook this dish. You could replace the oxtails with eggplant or whole pre-cooked mushrooms.

Preparation time
15 minutes

Cooking time
3 hours 30 minutes

Servings
6 Servings

Ingredients

- 1 pint red wine
- 3 1/4 lbs. oxtail
- 2 1/2 lbs. carrots
- 1 bunch spring onions
- 1 bouquet of thyme and bay leaves
- 3 tbsp. olive oil
- 1 oz. butter
- Salt
- Pepper

Preparation

Step 1: At the supermarket, ask your butcher to cut the meat for you to make your cooking easier. Most supermarkets have it cut and packaged.

Step 2: Peel the carrots and onions. Cut the carrots into slices.

Step 3: Heat the butter and the oil in a pot. Add the meat and brown it all over. Next, add the onions and the bouquet of thyme and bay leaves, and season with salt and pepper.

Step 4: Pour the wine in the pot and bring to a boil.

Step 5: Reduce the heat, cover the pot, and cook gently for a further 2-1/2 hours on low heat.

Step6: Add the carrots and cook for another 45 minutes.

Step7: Place the meat in a dish, pour on the cooking juices, and add the carrots.

Step 8: Serve immediately.

Salmon and Green Tomatoes Club Sandwich

This is a typical sandwich. It includes all you need to enrich your nutrition. If you are having this particular dish for lunch, a chardonnay white wine should be your first choice. This is a summer dish, but can be prepared all year long.

Preparation time
15 minutes

Cooking time
None

Servings
6 Servings

Ingredients

- 3 green tomatoes
- 18 slices of whole wheat bread
- 2 hard-boiled eggs
- 2 tbsp. lemon dressing
- 1 clove garlic
- 6 slices smoked salmon
- A few slices of cucumber
- Olive oil
- Salt
- Pepper
- Fromage frais or crème cheese (fromage frais is recommended because it is much lower in fat)

Preparation

Step 1: Wash, dry, and cut the tomatoes in two and then into thin semi-circles.

Step 2: Shell and fine-chop the hard-boiled eggs; stir them into the lemon dressing

Step 3: Peel and chop the garlic, and mix it with salt and pepper.

Step 4: Lightly toast the slices of whole-wheat bread.

Step 5: Spread the egg mixture on six slices of bread and top them with the green tomatoes. Spread six other slices of bread with the cheese and top them with a slice of smoked salmon. Place this slice on top of the other one, and cover with the remaining slice. Push down gently on the top of the sandwich to press it together; cut it in two diagonally. Keep it in place with a wooden cocktail stick decorated with the cucumber slices, and serve right away.

Useful Tips: If you are a vegetarian, remove some of the ingredients and add vegetables like spinach and beans. It will have almost the same taste as the one with meat and dairy.

Scallops with Baby Vegetables

This dish is a bit expensive to prepare, but you could get your vegetables from your favorite farmers market and the scallops from your nearest Asian supermarket. It is much cheaper when doing it this way. This is a very delicate dish and contains most of the vitamins that your body requires.

Preparation time
20 minutes

Cooking time
20 minutes

Servings
6 Servings

Ingredients

- 1 zucchini
- 6 scallops
- 2 carrots
- 5 oz. fresh shelled peas
- 2 tbsp. olive oil
- 1/2 pint vegetable stock
- Freshly ground white pepper
- 1/4 stick salted butter
- 1 shallot (purple onion)
- 2 sprigs parsley
- Sea salt
- Rock salt

Preparation

Step 1: Make a bed of rock salt on each of the six serving plates. Place the six empty scallop shells on each plate and place them aside.

Step 2: Wash, dry, and pluck the parsley. Finely chop it.

Step 3: Wash the zucchini and the peas. Peel the carrots. Finely dice the zucchini and the carrots. Peel and chop the shallot.

Step 4: Gently heat the olive oil in a skillet. Fry the shallot for three minutes without it browning. Stir frequently. Add the diced carrots and fry for 2 minutes. Add the peas and pour on the vegetable stock. Lightly salt and season with pepper. Bring to a boil and cook for 10 minutes, then add the diced zucchini and cook for a further 5 minutes.

Step 5: Meanwhile, melt the butter in a frying pan and briskly fry the scallops. Season the mixture with salt and pepper and sprinkle with parsley. Distribute the vegetables and the cooking stock among the scallop shells. Add the scallops and serve immediately.

Useful Tips: You can also serve the vegetables and the scallops in a glass.

Desserts and Celebratory Drinks

Having a healthy drink contributes to a healthier body. Apart from water, you can make some drinks at home with friends and family to avoid being tempted to consume unhealthy drinks that will add extra pounds. I have chosen some drinks that are easier to make and fun when you are with company. I sincerely hope you enjoy them!

Singapore Sling Cocktail

Make this juice as a reward for your hard work. It is very easy to make in less than 10 minutes. It is perfect for all seasons. Have this drink in moderation, as it contains alcohol. Have it during or after a meal.

Preparation time
5 minutes

Cooking time
None

Servings
6 Servings

Ingredients

- 4 fl. oz. cherry liqueur
- 8 fl. oz. gin
- 2 fl. oz. grenadine syrup
- 6 fl. oz. lemon juice
- Mint
- Candied cherries
- Lemon slices

Preparation

Step 1: Pour all the ingredients straight into a glass, one after the other, in the following order: cherry, liqueur, gin, lemon juice, grenadine syrup.

Step 2: Decorate with a half-moon of lemon, candied cherries, and the mint leaves.

Red Currant Cocktail

This is a liqueur drink and should be consumed in moderation. Have this drink in a group and avoid making it in larger quantities.

Preparation time
5 minutes

Cooking time
None

Servings
6 Servings

Ingredients

- 1 pint white wine
- 4 fl. oz. peach liqueur
- 6 bundles redcurrants
- 6 mint leaves

Preparation

Step 1: Divide the liqueur among six champagne glasses and pour the wine over the top. Add a handful of redcurrants and a mint leaf to each glass.

Step 2: Serve chilled.

Pizza with Peaches and Apricot

This simple recipe is mostly prepared in the summer. The point price of the ingredients is affordable.

Preparation time
15 minutes

Cooking time
20 minutes

Servings
6 Servings

Ingredients

- 3 rolls pizza base pastry
- 5 peaches
- 9 apricots
- 9 small sprigs lemon thyme or mint (alternative)
- 5 packages of sweetener or honey (alternative)
- 1 tbsp. ground vanilla
- 2 tbsp. poppy seeds

Preparation

Step 1: Preheat the oven to 350ºF.

Step 2: Roll out the pastry as thin as possible and cut out eight small discs. Place them on a baking tray covered with a baking parchment.

Step 3: Wash the peaches and cut them into four pieces each. Remove the stones; cut the remaining peach into thin slices. Stone the apricots and cut them into four pieces each.

Step 4: Arrange the apricots and peaches on the pizza bases. Sprinkle the sweetener or honey, vanilla, and poppy seeds. Place them in the oven and let cook for 15-20 minutes.

Step 5: Serve straight from the oven, decorated with sprigs of lemon thyme.

Pears Poached in Red Wine

This dessert is the best of all! Not only do you receive the benefits of red wine, but you also smell and taste the fruit as well. Pears in this recipe can be exchanged with apples, and you will get the same results. Pears Poached in Red Wine is easy to make and low in cost. Do not serve it to anyone under the age of 21!

Preparation time
1 day 15 minutes

Cooking time
45 minutes

Servings
6 Servings

Ingredients

- 5 oz. sugar or 2 tbsp. honey
- 2 vanilla beans
- 3 sticks cinnamon
- 2 cloves
- 6 pears
- 1 pint red wine (low alcohol percentage)
- 1 star anise
- Cinnamon cookies (optional)

Preparation

Step 1: Cut the vanilla beans in two lengthwise and place in a pan with the red wine, sugar or honey, and spices. Bring to a boil.

Step 2: Meanwhile, peel the pears. When the wine starts to bubble, place the pears in the pan.

Step 3: Cook for 45 minutes on low heat, regularly dousing the pears with the wine. When the cooking time is up, lay the pears in a dish and totally cover with the wine sauce. Leave to cool and refrigerate until the following day.

Step 4: The next day, when you are ready to serve, place the pears in dessert bowls and pour the spicy wine over them.

Step 5: Serve chilled, accompanied by cinnamon cookies.

Peaches with White Wine and Lavender

As good as this recipe is, it should be consumed in moderation and should not be served to children under-twenty one! It is delicious, easy to prepare, and cheap. Most enjoy this dish in warm weather, but it is up to you to choose when to consume it. My mother usually prepares this dish during the holidays, and her guests really enjoy it. Have fun with this dish and lose weight while having fun in the kitchen!

Preparation time
15 minutes

Cooking time
25 minutes

Servings
6 Servings

Ingredients

- 1 pint white wine (low alcohol percentage)
- 1/2 cup sugar or 2 tbsp. honey
- 6 white peaches
- 1 tablespoon lavender flowers

Preparation

Step 1: Heat the wine, sugar or honey, and lavender flowers in a heavy-bottomed pan. Simmer for 10 minutes over low heat.

Step 2: Meanwhile, submerge the peaches for in boiling water for 10 seconds, and then refresh in a bowl of cold water. Peel them and cover them in lemon juice to prevent them from browning. Add them, one by one, to the simmering wine. Bring back to a boil, partially cover them, and gently simmer for a further ten minutes.

Step 3: When the cooking time is up, leave the peaches to cool in their juice and then cover them and place in the refrigerator until you are ready to serve. Serve them chilled with a few lavender flowers as decoration.

Section Three

The Mechanism of Fitness

To properly lose weight and stay fit, you must have a good fitness routine. This section illustrates how to introduce a fitness routine into your daily life and how to make it work. There are some illustrations of different poses and aspects of a great workout to put in great use.

Chapter Seven

The Art of Physical Fitness

Tips for a Healthy Fitness Routine

Good nutrition is not the only way to achieve a great body and health. Fitness could help increase your overall body endurance, life expectancy, and promote good health. All it requires is just a few hours of physical exercises each week. Exercising releases proteins and strengthens your brain's neurons and cells. The brain's neurons and cells are directly related to your learning and memory abilities; therefore, taking good care of your brain is essential. There are pros and cons in any activities we partake in. The disadvantage of fitness is that it takes some time and requires a weekly schedule and a great amount of motivation to see results. The advantage is the good health, the fun, and the augmentation of your life expectancy, as previously mentioned. The following tips will help you find the right exercise and advice to help beginners with their exercise routines.

Have Proper Nutrition

Make sure you are eating enough food to support the new muscle growth. Many people struggle with food insufficiency to support the kind of growth they are trying to achieve. Do not forget to eat plenty of carbs, which are especially important for muscle builders. By that, I am referring to healthy fats, such as avocado, olive oil etc. To get enough energy to work out, you will need a variety of proteins, carbs, and healthy fats, such as Omega-3s. Aim for 45% proteins, 35% carbohydrates, and 20% fat.

If you are not consuming proteins at every meal, you will be missing an opportunity to build your muscles, and it might take you a longer time to see improvement. If your body runs short on glucose after hard workouts, your body then uses muscle tissue for protein and carbohydrates, undoing your hard work; therefore, stay away from low-carb diets, and eat an appropriate amount of carbs given the intensity of your workouts, but wait a couple of hours before working out or it might upset your stomach. Do not exercise on an empty stomach. It is best to eat a healthy carbohydrate 30-60 minutes before exercising. Some great ideas for pre-workout snacks are yogurt and fruit, a small bowl of oatmeal, or a banana.

Fitness Tips

- An exercise journal will help you get started and keep you motivated to move into new fitness programs. You may think that it is easier to keep track in your head, but a diary is much better and will help you track your continued progress. Take this task, as well as your goal of achieving better fitness, seriously and give them the attention they deserve.
- Cleaning out your home or your car is also considered good exercise. Such exercise burns a great deal of calories. In addition to that, it is recommended to set up a regular time for physical exercises; in other words, keep your body active by doing highly intensive activities. Archery can be a way for one to work on fitness while having fun and learning a new skill at the same time. The repetitive drawing of the bow string works one's upper body. Drawing with each arm ensures that both sides get exercised. You can use common household items as weights without ever going to the gym. Milk jugs make fabulous weights for lifting. Hold a jug in each hand and do lunges down the hall. You can also consider lifting a jug repeatedly over your head or from your side to straight out. By performing this activity, you will start building up more strength over time.
- You should choose exercises adapted to your level. You have to understand that the average person cannot train like a professional bodybuilder. Be realistic about your body type and health to

develop a routine that will not exhaust you or damage your muscles. As you progress, you will be able to transform your routine. As you become more experienced in working out, it's very important that you make sure you adjust the amount of weight you lift. Once you get stronger, you are either going to have to increase your weight or your reps in order to get that pump you need for achieving additional muscle growth. Increasing your weight gradually protects you from overexerting yourself. If you are just starting to get in shape, you should not work out more than twice a week. This will give enough time for your muscles to heal and expand. As you get more experienced, add a third session every week.

- Find something that helps you stay motivated. Do not expect to have an entirely different body type within a few weeks; building muscles takes months, even years. You should set a list of realistic goals for yourself and learn patience. You will fail if you expect too much from your body. In case you are not seeing a difference after a few weeks of intensive training, measure your body fat. Perhaps your fat is slowly transforming into muscle, so you are not seeing a difference in your weight. This is a good thing: Once your body fat is reduced, you will be able to build muscles. I suggest you purchase exercise machines to use at home if you can afford them. This purchase will be a motivation to perform to the best of your ability. To start off, shop around for the best deals and search for available store coupons to save even more. Be sure to choose quality pieces that will last for a long period of time.
- Stay well hydrated when you want to stay healthy and exercise more. About two hours before your workout session, consume about two servings (one serving is 8 oz.) of water; during your workout, you should drink at least 5 oz. for every 20 minutes of exercising. Dehydration can cause some negative effects on the body and can lead to hospitalization in severe cases.
- Rock climbing is a great way to increase your fitness level. For this exercise, all you will need are a good pair of shoes that fit tightly and a rock or a wall to climb. This is an excellent exercise routine

that works out your whole body, as it targets all the muscle groups in your body.

- In case you are looking for a gym for weight training, choose the one that you will enjoy the most and take a tour before signing up. During your tour, check to see if there are loose weights lying on the floor. If that were the case, it should be an alarm that the gym rarely gets cleaned up, either by the clients or by the management; therefore, keep on shopping around for a cleaner and more organized gym to reduce your risk of injuries or diseases. More importantly, keep fitness costs to a minimum by researching free or low-cost ways to stay fit. Walking, jogging, and running are all great ways to get fit. There are free online workout videos and some television programs that may be beneficial without breaking the bank.

- In case you need a gadget, an outfit or any other fitness related needs, Target, Marshall, or any other discounted outlets would have it a discounted price. When exercising daily, keeping your music track list repetitive causes boredom; therefore, update your tracks weekly to spice up your new routine. Furthermore, to help your fitness commitment last more than a month, budget $50 for some portable music device to assist you with your workouts.

- Plan out your routine properly! It is a good idea to work on only one or two specific muscle groups per day instead of jumping around. By doing this, you will be able to give your muscles enough time to rest before putting them through another really exhausting workout session. Your muscles need some time to heal, so just give them time.

- Whenever you are working out, flex your arms for maximum benefits especially while doing arm curls. Start by doing a standard arm curl, but make sure it is completely straight. Perform the exercise by flexing your triceps at the end of your repetitions. This technique works out your arm muscles by using their entire range of motion. During your workout, some soreness is normal, but pain is not. When this happens, stop immediately and take a break before resuming. If the pain does not subside for a day or two, head to the doctor, as you may have a severe injury. Do not do your normal exercise routine when you are feeling under the weather. It is better to go easy on your body by giving it time to heal and recuperate. Take the day off and allow the body to use its resources to heal the sickness, not build muscles. The older you get, the less flexible your muscles are, which increases the risk of muscle pains. If you are younger than 40, you should try to hold each stretching position for at least 30 seconds. After 40, increase the holding time to a full minute. This will keep your muscles pliable and strain-free.

- If you get cold feet about the idea of spending 30 minutes on a treadmill, you might want to give a hula hoop a try as your fitness routine. As you are rotating your hips, bend at the knees slightly. This will keep the hoop aloft, while burning extra calories and target problem areas like love handles.

- Keep in mind that muscles don't grow while you're working out; they grow during the resting period when they feel sore. For this reason, it's most efficient to alternate workout days to give your muscles time to rest and grow. Working out heavily every single day will just wear your muscles down. Therefore, knowing the best basic exercises for muscle building will give you fast-track results. Be sure to include squats, dead lifts, and bench presses to maximize your use of time and energy. These muscle-building techniques will strengthen and build your muscles rapidly. Incorporate them into your regular routine and increase the number of repetitions you do in safe increments.

- Lastly, do not be afraid to ask for help at the gym. In case you are unaware of how to utilize a machine, go ahead and seek help from the staff. Understand how to use both aerobic and strength-building equipment. Asking for help will give you the confidence to actually use the equipment. The more comfortable you are in your workout environment, the more you will keep up with your workouts. To achieve greater weight-loss results and be well-fit, the first thing to do is to maximize your workouts. The more exercise you can bear in a shorter period of time, the better your weight loss results will be. Make your exercises "denser" by shortening your breaks in-between intervals or removing your breaks altogether between your routines. You will see improved results if you apply this for a period of time.

In case you are uncomfortable working out in public, I have illustrated a workout routine at the end of the book for your use. As you can see, building muscle safety is something you accomplish with some knowledge and common sense. Applying these tips rather than a dangerous fad workout will give you the best chance to succeed in building a body you can be proud of. Soon you will be looking and feeling great! These fitness tips should inspire you enough to take fitness efforts seriously. Now that your goals are in sight, all you need is to stick to your plan. Good luck on your program!

Daily Workouts Instructions

Exercising

Many want to get themselves in good shape; however, they believe that it is just too difficult to achieve. One thing to keep in mind is *education*. Educating yourself on how to become fit is the best way to start. Use what you will be learning here and move forward.

Set up a workout routine. Get up 20 minutes early, but avoid a hardcore workout at first. Warm up by doing some aerobic exercises or jump rope. Doing your workouts when you first get up in the morning helps make your day more productive.

- Employ your friends to do some fitness regimens with you if you are not sticking to it. Exercising with company could be a source of motivation to achieve your goals. Having an exercise partner can foster a beneficial sense of competition, which may push you to work even harder than you normally would by yourself.
- Variety is important when it comes to exercising. If you go through the same exercise routines every single day, you will be more likely to give up out of boredom. As your body becomes used to repetitive exercises, it spends less energy accomplishing each

routine, and you will begin to notice fewer results. Introduce new exercises as often as you can to help keep things fun and fresh each time you exercise.

- When working out, you should have a specific sequence to the exercises. To start, use dumbbells first, then the barbells, and lastly the machines. Workout coaches say that smaller muscles in our body experience tiredness before larger muscles; therefore, it is a great idea to begin with the dumbbells first. As you enervate certain muscles in your body, you should change to a workout that requires less effort to work out the smaller muscle groups.
- Walking can help you attain the fitness goals that you desire. You can walk using the heel-to-toe method by walking on your heel first and then moving all the way to your toes. This helps your calves to work out harder and works out your whole body. Try to work your arms as well when walking. All you need to do is to bend the elbows by swinging your arms with each step you take.
- Avoid bouncing while stretching. This action usually puts undue strain on your muscles, and it is not beneficial to your flexibility to bounce when you stretch. As a matter of fact, doing so is an invitation to injuries. Be stable, stretch the best you can, and avoid the bouncy activities.
- A stability ball is a good option for good exercise, assuming you will be able to utilize it without any complications. Your core muscles will be toned up, as they will help maintain your posture and your overall balance from this simple change. You can also use the ball to perform other fitness exercises, such as wall squats.
- Laying out some specific fitness goals is the best way to jumpstart your motivation. Making a goal can help you dodge some obstacles, rather than becoming fixated on them. Setting goals can keep you working steadily if you think of them as part of your continuing process that you will always strive toward.

There is no other feeling in the world like the feeling of health and fitness. Most people feel overwhelmed because they lack exercise, but now you can begin a new change by following the right tips and advice. Practice the suggested tips that you have read, and you can easily reach your goals, making physical exercises more enjoyable and easier to master.

Types of Physical Exercises

Cardiovascular Exercises

Whenever you sign up for a fitness program, it is important that you consume enough protein to help your body build up muscles. Start by selecting lean protein sources for an easy way to increase your protein consumption. Without enough proteins in your diet, you will have difficulties achieving the benefits of your workouts. Cardiovascular exercises are phenomenal for building and strengthening muscles. Make sure you have your protein intake daily to ease your way into the fitness world. Below are some low-key cardiovascular activities that you can perform to reap maximum benefits and lose weight faster and easier.

Aerobic Exercises

Spinning classes can be a fun way to get in shape. Many people go to the gym deciding that they solely want to focus on aerobic exercise to shed pounds, but give up down the road. Well, spinning is one of the best ways to lose weight, as it removes the total amount of stress on your joints that you might get from long-distance running, while still pairing you with a calorie-burning cardiovascular activity.

Running

There is no key to success in fitness more than performing regular workouts. An undemanding solution is to find a cardiovascular activity that you find enjoyable. Running is an inexpensive and easy way to get fit without the burden of high monthly payments. It works out your whole body, even your love handles. All you need is some good running shoes and you are ready to hit the pavement. The most crucial way to see regular results is to perform a cardiovascular exercise as often as possible. First, purchase a quality pair of running shoes that fit you accurately. If your shoes do not fit, your running program will never feel fun and comfortable, so getting a top-quality shoe will save you money in the future due to their longevity. To start your running activity, divide your total run into three separate periods. For the first period, keep your running speed just above your personal minimum. The second period consists of increasing your speed to a medium pace. The third period is about increasing your speed to the fastest you can. A great fitness tip for runners who experience sore calves would be to sleep on your belly and let your feet dangle off the bed. Over the course of the night, your calves will stretch out just from being in that position. Stretching, warming up, and cooling down are also great ways to assist you with these calf pains.

Second, whenever you are running short distances, go faster than you normally would for a long distance. Doing this will improve your running form and make your muscles less susceptible to injuries. When running longer distances, it is important to run at a steady pace. Sometimes, running too fast for long distances can cause injuries and potential leg pains that can keep you off of the track for a long period. During your run, practice inhaling in a way that your stomach rises as you do so. By doing this, you are making sure that your lungs are fully filling with oxygen, which helps increase your endurance. The best way to practice is to lie on the floor with a book on your belly. Then practice pushing the book up when inhaling. This will make a difference in your running routine and flatten your stomach as well. Another abdominal workout is called vacuum. Vacuum is basically sucking or pulling your belly button toward your spine and holding it there for 10 seconds while maintaining your normal breathing pattern. This process works your transversus muscles and will flatten and slim your waistline. When running, breathe with your belly for maximum performance. When you exhale, your stomach should be tucked in tight, whereas on the inhale, it should expand out. This form of breathing engages the diaphragm and lets you make use of your total lung capacity. This technique improves your endurance and your breathing efficiency.

Third, utilize the full potential of your legs, as well as the rest of the body, to maximize your amount of oxygen. You can strengthen your legs with isotonic exercise. Many sports, such as basketball, cycling, footballs, and running, require strong legs. Isotonic exercise is a tense workout that contracts a muscle for a certain amount of time, and if done regularly, great muscles will build up. Weight lifting is a particularly good example of this exercise, as it helps develop and tone your muscles, and bests of all, increase your joint flexibility (very beneficial for your golden age).

The art of fitness is one that can be enjoyed by nearly everyone. Most who find it difficult are the ones who are having trouble finding which physical exercise they enjoy the most. There are thousands and thousands of videos that you can use online for your own workout enjoyment. If you are having difficulties staying active, think about including your dogs in your fitness routine. Maybe you have not noticed, but dogs tend to light up your day and they love staying active, so the best way to work out or help them stay fit is to run with them. Dogs love running, and by being with them, you will pick up their energy and remind yourself that you could also enjoy running as well as your best friend. To make things handy and a little easier, I have illustrated some workouts that you could use, including those of leg-muscle building. Get serious and get into your own personal routine every chance you get. Now that you have more fitness knowledge to add to your bag of tricks, you can easily become a healthier person and build stronger muscles.

Note: In a cold weather, make sure you warm up your body with a short bout of running to boost your heart and buffer your joints before your normal routine. This technique reduces injuries and gives you much pleasure in your running routine.

Swimming Aerobics

In case you are putting off fitness exercises due to your dislike of sweat, swimming could be your best option. Whenever reaching your fitness goal is hindered by your excess weight or joint problems, try water aerobic exercises. Your swimming pool could be used as a gym. As a result, you reduce your body fat, burn extra calories, and build lean muscles without putting extra pressure on your joints. Most franchise fitness clubs have a swimming pool, so take advantage. Swimming, as I mentioned, is low-impact exercise, and most people end up having a lot of fun once they are in the pool. The water keeps your body revitalized and cools your body during your workout, and best of all is the lack of sweat during your routine. In order to get the most out of your fitness routine when swimming, be sure to work your ankles' flexibility. That prevents you from unnecessary injuries and increases your performance in the water. This can be done simply by suspending your legs and pointing your toes away from you, then upward for a full minute. Before plunging into the water and swimming, spend some time ducking your head and body in and out of the water. Breathe in while you are on the surface, and try to breathe out while you are under. This small tip give you time to acclimatize to the water and increase your enjoyment of swimming.

Now that you have gained some knowledge, it is time to set a schedule and stick to it. Start slowly and add new exercises to your routine as you move on. Take your time, avoid over-exhaustion, and most important, have a good time. These three elements are the basics of a great start in the world of fitness.

Walking

Everywhere you turn, you will notice new recommendations to incorporate exercise into your life. Know that you do not need a gym to get the benefits of exercising. Take a walk as often as you can to improve your blood circulation, strengthen your body, and burn calories. Walking is an excellent technique to stay in shape and tone your body.

Useful Techniques for Walking

Design your fitness plan and avoid injuries. This means using good posture and form while working out with equipment and skipping a day after each session. Replace your sneakers every few hundred miles to avoid leg injuries and improve stability if you walk a lot for a workout routine. Take your workout outside instead of walking on your treadmill. Not only is fresh air better for your body and you will have better scenery, but going outside is a boost to your workout. Starting an appropriate level of fitness improves your rate of workouts. Begin by walking around the block a few days each week. After a week, lengthen your walk by a block or two. You will find that you will enjoy your physical activities more after a week of lengthening your walk and adding a block or two to your routine. Purchase a pedometer to track your steps each time you go for a walk. It can be a great investment if you are serious about losing weight by walking and dieting. A pedometer, a fitbit or your smartphone racks the number of steps you take, and best of all, they tend to be affordable and are easily found online and in stores. Make sure that you are taking at least 10,000 steps a day if you dislike cardiovascular exercises. For more exercise, try adding more activities into everything you do. Walking to a farther water fountain or restroom at work will increase the number of steps you take in a day, and walking a little faster when going up the stairs or simply walking across a parking lot can add intensity to those steps.

I am sure you are confident enough to enjoy your fitness journey. Use these instructions and suggestions wisely as a starting point; you can be in the best shape of your life. You will not only look better, but you also will feel better and have more energy than ever. before.

Yoga

No matter what your personal fitness goals are currently, there is always room for more improvement. Luckily, there are efficient ways for you to get your fitness routines done with total satisfaction. Yoga is an ancient workout that many are aware of but do not act on. Not only does yoga give you a complete workout, it also improves your overall flexibility. It is mostly recommended for muscle builders. Yoga is not a feminine type of workout; it is for everyone. Most individuals wonder if using yoga as a fitness routine will provide muscle strength and not just flexibility. The answer to this question is that it indeed does provide muscle strength. It does so in a way that weight training on machines does not; it is all about using your own body weight to train the muscles, particularly the support muscles when you struggle to maintain proper balance in a pose. Holding a pose for longer than you have previously done will provide even more strength. Many fitness experts claim that one of the most pervasive workout myths is "no pain, no gain." There are plenty of low-intensity exercise techniques that can keep you fit and healthy. Those include yoga, light stretching, and walking. Hatha yoga's sun salutation practice is an excellent path to great fitness. By performing this type of yoga, anyone can enjoy 15 or 30 minutes of gentle stretching, deep breathing, and quiet focus every day. This physical form of yoga relaxes the mind, strengthens and stretches the muscles, and loosens the joints. Perform the hatha yoga sun salutation first thing in the morning and just before bed, and you will notice a great improvement in your mood and your fitness level.

Now that you aware of yoga's benefits, you are ready to make a difference and feel healthier every day. I hope that what you have read above encourages you to get started today! There is always room for improvements. Seeing improvements will only inspire you to work harder. Now is the time to take action and enjoy your workout!

Muscles Building Techniques

A fitness routine is about more than just getting healthy. Getting fit improves your lifestyle and your overall satisfaction in many ways. It can give you more energy, provide an enjoyable hobby and even help you live longer. Your fitness routine can always benefit from a little novelty. Below are some ideas you might consider adding into your new regimen.

When working out, do not forget to exercise your arms as well, especially for muscle building. A good fitness tip for building up your arms is to work the opposite muscles in opposite sets to each other. The best example would be to work the triceps and then follow with the biceps. Give each one of them the opportunity to rest while the other picks up the work. This minimizes your workout time and maximizes the intensity of your exercise. For large arms, perform bicep curls and triceps extensions. Biceps and triceps make up the majority of arm mass and can be easily worked out with curls and triceps extensions. Use preacher curls, an exercise where you hold a barbell very close to the middle of your chest and curl it as you would with a dumbbell, is very useful for establishing forearm strength as well. If you lift at the gym, the machine that you want may not always be available. When these devices are in use, make sure to engage in another form of exercise to keep your body active at all times. Standing still should never be an option if you want to maximize your productivity. Whenever you are lifting weights that target your arms, it is generally a good idea to lift one arm at a time. Oftentimes, one arm is stronger than the other and can do more of the work whenever you lift with both arms at the same time. Exercises that isolate your arms will ensure that both get a proper workout. You can work out anywhere, whether at home or in your office; put your mind to work creatively. Working at a desk does not mean you cannot exercise! Take your 20 oz. water bottle as a weight to work on your triceps and biceps while on the phone with clients or checking your e-mails. You can build your calves and strengthen your knees just by doing seated leg lifts, or you can practice balancing on a sofa cushion to improve your body's overall balance. Stand on it with one leg, and move a medicine ball, jug, or something else a tad weight from one hand to the other, side to side, and behind your head. When you have this down, challenge yourself by doing it with your eyes closed. If you have a very demanding job and have no time and energy to get fit, these simple tricks could really turn your workplace into a mini-gym! If you are interested in becoming more fit, figure out creative ways to adapt to your surroundings. Although it may seem impossible at times, you can work out anywhere. Your home, the park, and the gym are all viable options. Think about what exercises work best in the different locations ahead of time, so you never have an excuse not to work out. As previously mentioned, finding a way to maintain your fitness goals can be difficult, but the right kind of information always helps take the pressure off your shoulders. There are many tips that can help you reach and maintain your goals; search and preserve them for your next fitness regimen. Use the small tips provided in this chapter to get on your way to becoming a fitness guru, living a more fulfilling and healthier life.

Simple Workouts

Stepping classes are an excellent way for women to get fit. This type of exercise can shape up the thighs and butt. It improves the best region to increase feminine beauty. Other exercises, such as body squats and lunges, can also help firm up these muscles. Because they provide a majority of the body's lifting capacity, trunk, core, and thigh muscles are essential to both genders. Lunges are a perfect exercise that works out your calf and thigh muscles. To perform them, simply stand with your left leg slightly in the front and your right leg slightly in the back. Next, lean forward with your left knee slightly bent. Lastly, stand back up. Perform this with each leg 10 times for three sets. One important aspect of weight you should always be aware of is that skinny never means fit; therefore, avoid making the mistake of believing that you are fit when in reality you are unfit and hurt your diet with poor nutritional provisions. True fitness comes through a proper diet and plenty of hard work. The recommendations mentioned will assist you in remaining healthy and fit for the rest of your life. If you follow the tips you have read above, you should be well on your way to actually becoming a fit individual in a short time.

Chapter Eight

Physical Exercise Illustrations

Office Workout

This is a quick exercise for individuals with a busy schedule. To start, use the stopwatch on your phone, watch or the Internet. It is important that you time yourself. This will help you know your body better and help you work out effectively in the comfort of your own home or office. The exercises are not only effective on your abs, but useful for the whole body as well. Expect some soreness the following day and drink a lot of fluid after the workout to reduce the risk of injuries.

Step (1): Position yourself as illustrated. Then move your legs forward and backward as if you were running in one place, but in a bent position. Perform this exercise for 30 seconds non-stop. Depending on your weight, you can start with 10 seconds and then increase the time. This exercise helps build abs and strengthen your shoulders.

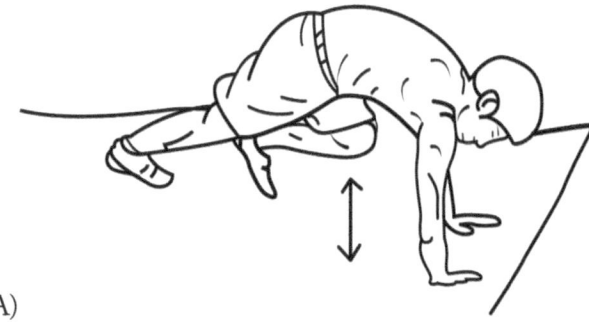

(A)

Step (2): Elbow Crunch

Put your hands behind your head and then raise your legs upward to a medium height, as seen in sketch (B). Lastly, lift your head with your hands still behind it forward toward your knees (C). Most importantly, keep your feet elevated! Hold this position for 30 seconds. Ten lifts should be enough for this exercise then move to the next.

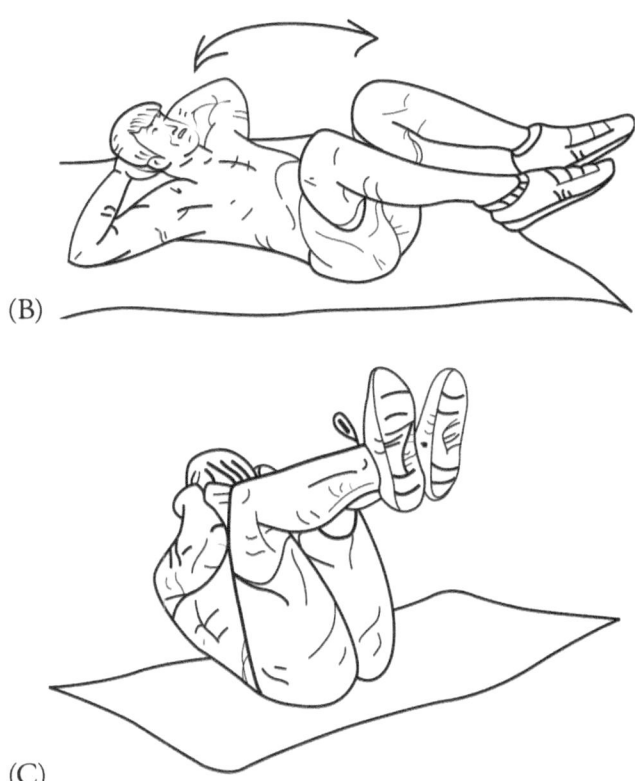

(B)

(C)

Step (3): Plank with Stretch

Stretch your whole body as illustrated for 10 seconds, and then repeat Step 1 for another 30 seconds. You should feel the burn at this point! If not, you are doing it wrong or taking too many breaks or too long of a break between the exercises.

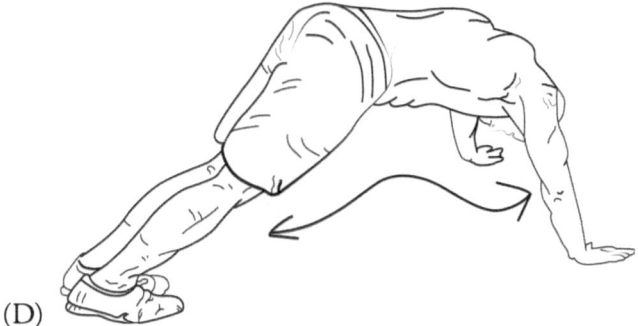

(D)

Leg Toning Pilates

These steps show quick results and only take 10-15 minutes of your time depending on how intensively you want to work out. I used to have cellulite, and these little tips saved me money and brought my cellulite to a minimum. Be patient with this exercise. It works progressively and as long as you keep it up, you will have no problem rocking your beautiful legs.

Step (1): Squat Kick Back

Stand up straight as in image (A) and try to sit down on an imaginary chair (B); then draw yourself back up and extend your right leg backward as seen in image (C). Then switch to the other leg. Four to six times on each leg should be enough, but increase it gradually as your body gets used to it.

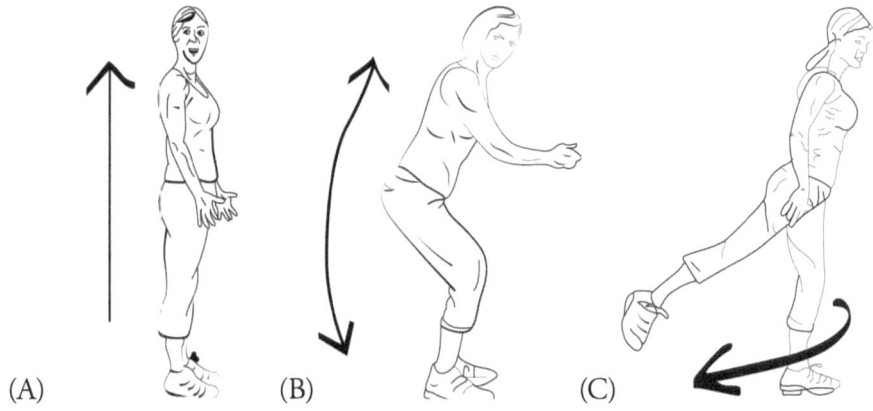

(A)   (B)   (C)

Step (2): Plier Sweep Exercise

This exercise is great for tightening up the thighs as well as your butt and abs. Spread your legs widely, as seen as in image (D), and keeping your abs as tight as you can, drop down onto your knees. As you come back up, sweep your leg across as if you were kicking a ball in front of you, as in image (E). Do so 10 times by switching sides, meaning five sweeps on each side. Make it as smooth as possible. In case you can't get completely down, try to make it as far as you can, and progressively challenge yourself!

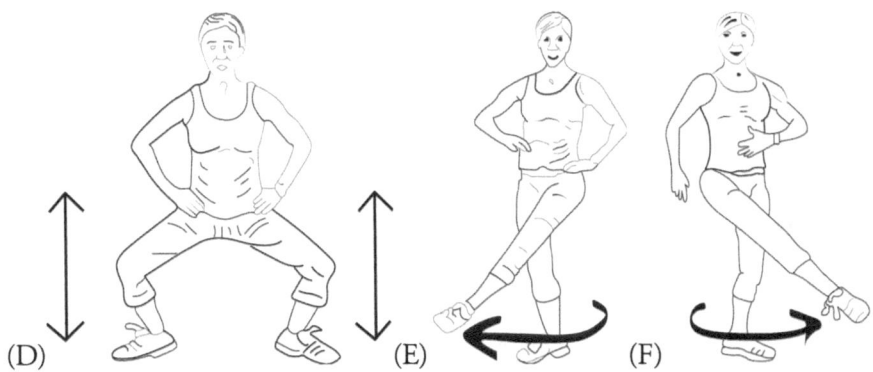

(D)   (E)   (F)

Step (3): Pass-Through Lunge

This exercise is a bit painful, but it is useful if you want to tone that body of yours. To start, take your foot forward as in image (G) and come down into a complete full-range motion. Make sure the back knee points down, then pull that leg through, balance it upward as in (H), and go into a reverse lunge. The back knee should point down, as shown in image (I). Then bring it up again and bring it forward as in image (G). Then go on again in a front lunge, back through, and back lunge. Perform about five on each side and switch. Perform these exercises regularly, and you will notice a more satisfying result at the end.

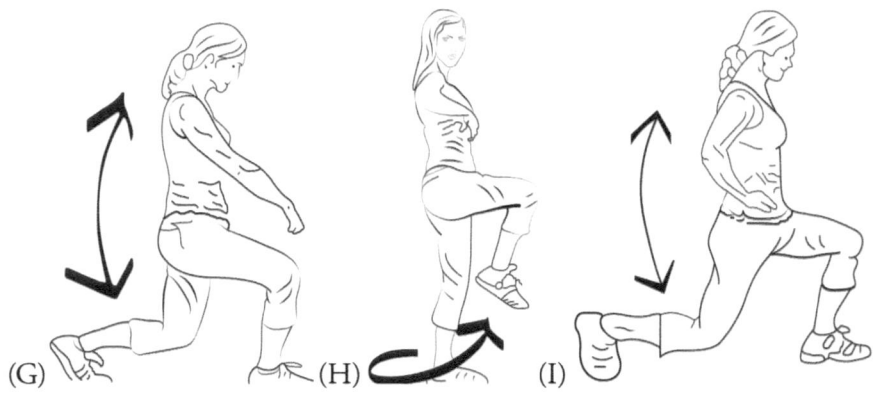

(G)   (H)   (I)

Step (4): Balance and Kick Exercises

Lock your abs completely tight, then take your right foot and bring it behind, as in (L); be mindful of your left knee; it should be as straight as possible. Then bring your right leg forward and kick it to the side. Try it again, this time a little faster, "down and up," "down and up." Perform this four times on each side. Increase to 10 or more depending on what you can take. Breathe and relax your body while doing this, and then try the other side.

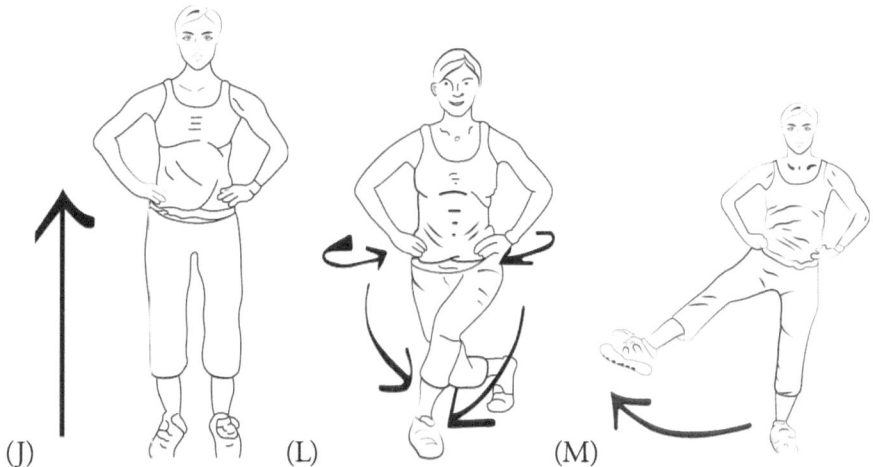

(J)   (L)   (M)

Step (5): Abs and Abdominal Stretch

Sit as in image (N) on your carpet or yoga mat. Make sure your feet are lined up next to each other, then lie on your back as in (O), with your hands relaxed to the sides. Next, tighten your abs as you lift your body up as in image (P). You will feel the stretch in your legs and back; then lower your body down and repeat the movement again. Make sure you drop down carefully, and as you drop your body, don't let it drop down to the floor of its own weight; lift it up and down, then squeeze up and down. Four times on each side should be enough. gradually increase it as you progress, but most importantly, keep your hips steady east to west. This exercise gives you a complete abdominal workout. When you are done, come to a sitting position on your mat for the last exercise.

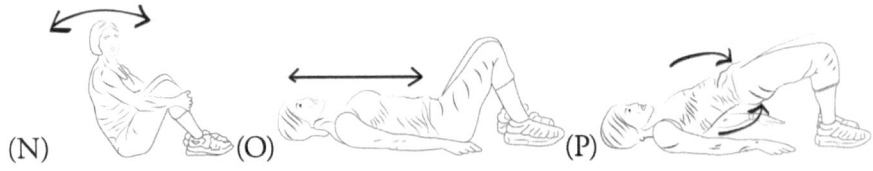

(N)   (O)   (P)

Step (6): The Bun Burn

For this exercise, you will surely feel the pain, but keep steady! Keep your abs tight with a nice long spine. Imagine that you are balancing a soccer ball on your back, then take your right knee toward your chest as in (R) and then shoot it back down keeping your hips parallel to the floor. Do that several times, and then do a leg lift just as in (S). Feel it, then curl it up as in image (T). I recommend you do this about 4-5 times on each side. Lift the knee up to your chest, then straight leg, and at last curl it up! Follow these three steps, and you will feel the burn; in case you don't, you are doing it the wrong way. For the last step, relax into a child pose to rest your body; and you are done!

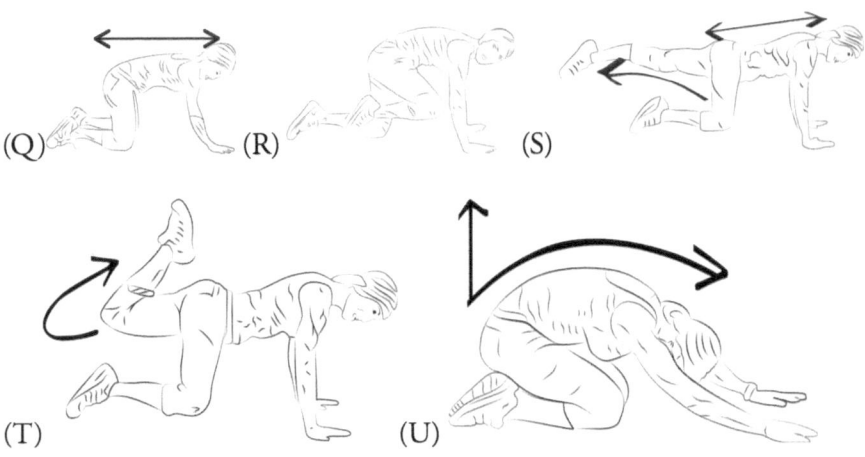

(Q)   (R)   (S)

(T)   (U)

Muffin Top Pilates

In case you are struggling with an unwanted muffin top, you are in luck; these exercises below are all you need. They could be performed daily or twice a week depending on what your body can take, but don't forget to pay a visit to your physician to find out if you are eligible for these workouts. For these exercises, all you need is a weight to hold and a yoga mat! The weight can be between 2-1/2 to 10 lbs. Please remember that this routine can be challenging and consume a lot of water to reduce soreness the following day.

Step (1): Oblique Twist

Cross your legs just like in the picture, but make sure you keep your heels on the floor if you are a beginner. In case you need a more core exercise routine to kill that muffin top faster, then cross your legs and lift them up (about 2 inches above the ground), make sure your elbows are stretched widely, and don't forget that you are holding a weight. Lean on your side until your elbows touch the Yoga mat just like in image (A) and come right up as in image (B) but make sure you don't let go of the weight. Perform this routine as long as you can for a beginner, but keep in mind that you will gradually increase the number of crunches you do weekly to see faster results.

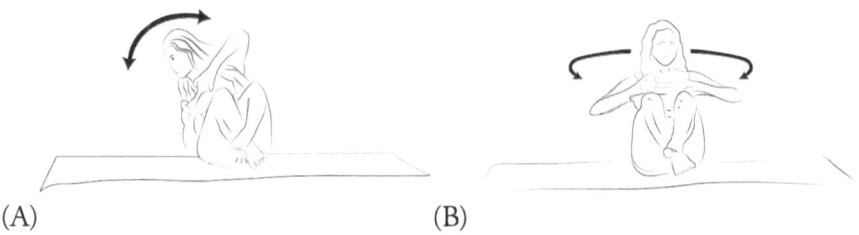

(A)   (B)

Step (2): Oblique Stretch

After Step 1, come completely on your knees and stretch your left leg completely straight to the side, then stretch your arms as a "plane." Then come down as in image (D), making sure your arm is parallel to your right leg, which is still kneeling. Avoid bending and be as straight as possible!

Then come right back up as in image (C). Perform these movements at least five times on the right side and five times on the left side, this time stretching your right leg.

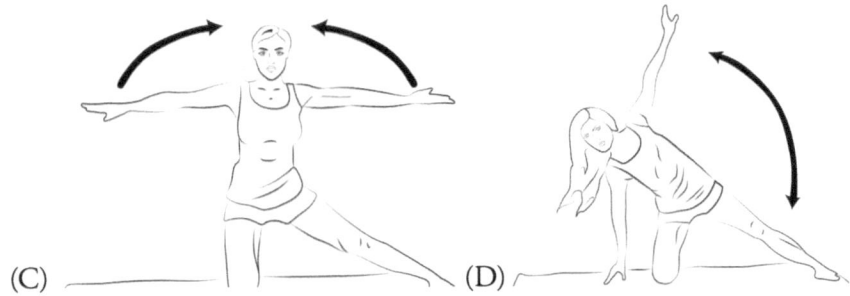

(C)   (D)

Step (3): Intense Oblique Workout

This step is an intense oblique workout exercise to burn most of the fat on your abdomen and tone your abs. First, bring both hands together over your head as shown in image (E). Lift up as straight as possible and come down on your right side, just like image (F), and then lift back up as shown in image (E). The important thing is to discourage yourself from quitting! It will be difficult at first, but keep at it if you want to say goodbye to those love handles. Try to perform it five times on each side, and gradually increase the number of repetition as you progress in your daily routine.

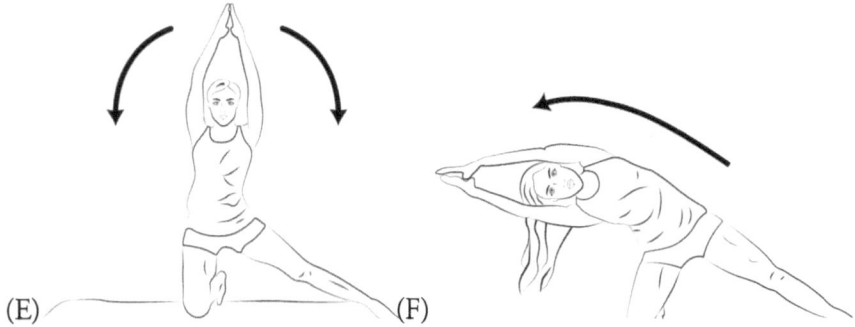

(E)   (F)

Try to perform these exercises at least 3-4 times weekly to see rapid results. Please do keep in mind that you will feel some soreness, which is normal after such intense routines, which is why drinking a lot of water helps.

5 Minute Office Workout

For those of you who do not have time to hit the gym or even workout at home, here is a quick five minutes workout for you. This is just four steps of exercises, but it is almost comparable to a full-body workout. As always, please consult your physician before doing anything for the first time. These exercises are great for de-stressing your body at the office; office work causes the muscles to be tight and ultimately weak, which is why doing these little exercises will help you achieve the toned and beautiful body you deserve. As I previously suggested, walking around or outside the office helps, but just in case you do not have time to get out, then follow these steps below.

Step (1): Start with hip flexes and the upper quad. To start, spread your leg then slowly, bend your left knee forward and straighten the other as seen in image (A). Stretch that back knee until you feel a great stretch down the front of your upper leg. Hold that pose for 30 seconds, and then move to the opposite side. Don't forget to breathe deeply through the nose instead of the mouth. Keep breathing and relax your muscles while you are performing the workout routine.

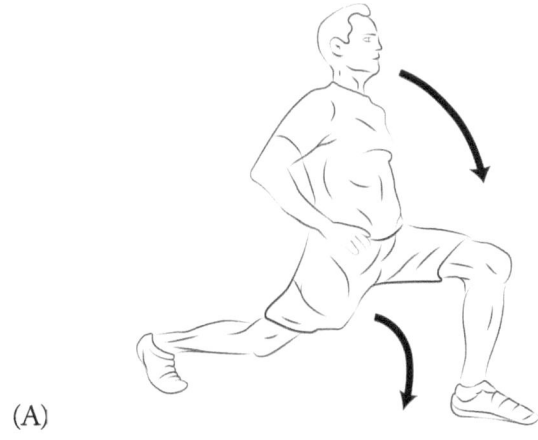

(A)

Step (2): Triceps Workout

Sit straight in your chair, then take one arm and bring it behind your head; follow with the opposite arm and grab the elbow as in image (B). Slightly pull. You should feel a burn, which is normal; it is good for this exercise. Hold that position for 30 seconds, and then move to the opposite side and hold that too for 30 seconds.

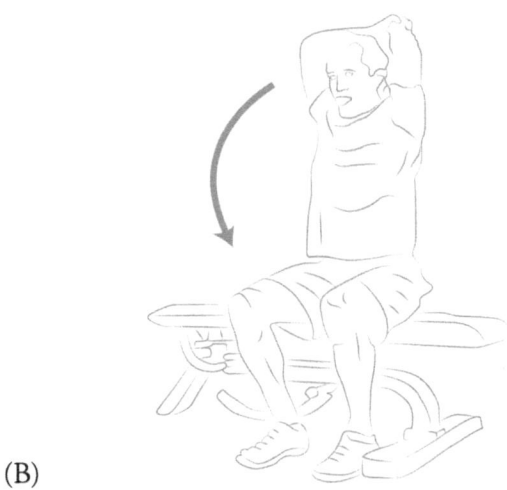

(B)

Step (3): Tight-Neck Workout

Again, sit up nice and tall in your chair and hold onto the side of your chair, as seen in image (C); then drop your ear toward the opposite shoulder until you feel some stretch in the neck. You can add more stretch by placing the opposite hand on your other ear and slightly pulling. Feel the burn and the stretch. Hold that pose for 30 seconds and switch sides. This stretch is powerful and will give you the toned muscles that you desire in the comfort of your own office. Have fun with it!

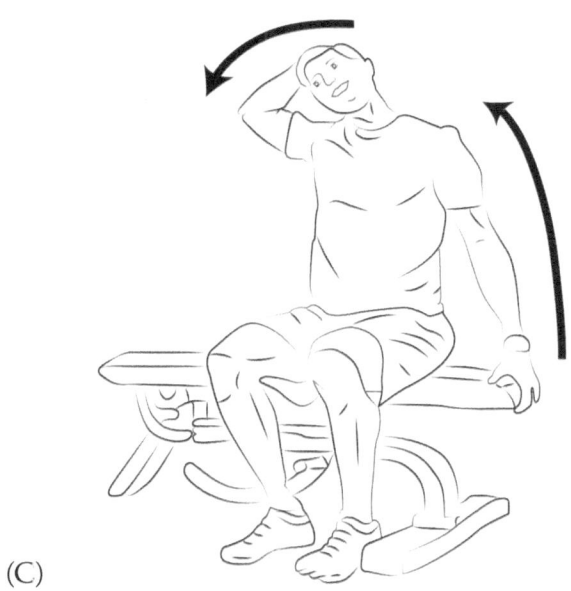

(C)

Chapter Nine

Eating Smartly

The Western diet has too much meat, lots of added fat and sugar causing more illnesses than we can bear. In reference to the to the nutrition paradigm that we have been discussing throughout this book, our best option to reinforce our immune systems and heal ourselves is through a healthy nutrition not through pills. Pills are created in a laboratory and you and I have no say in what goes in them, whereas in your kitchen, you have control over the ingredients. Every pill created has side effects which are inevitable. In the midst of our confusion and innocence about nutrition, it will be beneficial for us to step back, look at ourselves before choosing any unhealthy habit that will increase our risk of cardiovascular diseases, cancer, obesity, diabetes and others sicknesses associated with the Western diet. Junk foods, otherwise known as the refined foods, are the main cause of the Western illnesses that we experience. The best approach is to consume Whole Foods instead of the over-processed food that we find difficult to step away from. We only have one body and it cannot be replaced. It can definitely be healed by a doctor, but at what cost? I have met several individuals who were strongly against eating smartly. Their reasons are mainly about the cost but the question you should ask yourself is: Do I want to pay for it now or later? We always find excuses to avoid doing anything that is beneficial for us. Asking yourself "Do I want to pay for it now or later?" will push you to adapt to healthier choices. It is imperative that we prepare for the future now instead of focusing on our state of affairs in the future. Financial issues will always be there, but it is up to us to know which is important. That burger or that fried food that you are consuming will cause you more harm in the future than you have intended and at end, the only thing you will reap are regrets. We all know how much regret hurts. Gadgets will always be there, but your health can't wait! Have the *now or never* mentality. Figure out where to get your food locally. There are also thousands of farmers markets waiting to serve you. There are thousands of local farmers who also sell naturally raised meat or stone-grind flour. Find them and start getting your food from a natural source instead of chemically induced or refined foods that we do not seem to leave behind.

Limit your meat consumption

We have been taught that meat is good for us because of the proteins they contain. By now, we know that proteins do not only come from animals but also from plants. Red meat causes too many illnesses therefore; it is important that you step away from it or decrease your consumption to 3-6 oz. per week. The USDA recommends white meat over red meat but how often does a supermarket sell a naturally raised chicken or turkey? It is mostly loaded with hormones and antibiotics that we consume innocently. Start by halving your meat consumption, then reduce it to a minimum in a way that it becomes a treat not a daily food. My mother raised us differently than most families. Every condiment she uses except salt and seasonings came from a local farm. She befriended and built a strong relationship with the farmers and many of them brought their crops to us before anyone else. That was the joy of eating! Meat and dairy were only consumed once a week. She made sure that our allowance was limited and also befriended the cooks in our schools to monitor what went into our bodies. At the end of each week, usually Saturdays, we were in a fasting mood. Everything we ate on that day was juiced vegetables. My mother might seem like a *control freak* to you but I can honestly say she is the best mother I have ever known and I will forever be grateful for her input in my life. Since she is a professional chef, many would believe that we ate what we wanted but instead it was quite the opposite. This nutritional program that she opted for us limited our glorious days sick in bed. We were much stronger and healthier. Unfortunately, as an adult, I chose the opposite approach and consequently emptied my bank account at the end.

Before purchasing a food, make this checklist:

1. How far is really too far? Determine the boundaries of your local food. The USDA calls a food locally grown when it travels no more than 400 miles to our plates. By a food traveling that far, it loses some of its nutrients during the travel leaving us with fewer nutrients to heel ourselves.
2. Who supplies and distributes my food?
3. Who is my farmer and how is he or she been treated?
4. How much of the food I am about to purchase is distributed nationwide?
5. What food grows well in my region in the current season?
6. Who am I supporting by purchasing this particular food?

You control what goes into your mouth; it is up to you to determine what a healthy habit is. As a fellow meat lover, I understand how difficult it can be to reduce your meat consumption. Eating meat as a treat instead of a food has beneficial effects. All you need is to progressively reduce your meat consumption each week. Start by reducing it by 10% each week then another 10% and another until meat become a treat in your diet instead of a staple, but remember to get it from a natural source. You can also skip a day at a time or eat 10% smaller portions than you normally consumed. That alone will help you reduce your meat consumption to once a month instead of eliminating it completely all at once. We are creature of habits; we have to change one habit at a time. I usually shop for my meat at my local Whole Foods Market, where you have the option to discuss everything you need to know about your meat such as where it comes from and how it is raised. Oftentimes, there are also pamphlets at the store to illustrate where the ingredients have been produced or raised. Whole Foods Markets are not the only places you can acquire your meat. Always research your food before purchasing it. That will save you thousands of dollars in the long run. Always make yourself accountable for your actions. That mindset will not only put you on the right track, but also will keep you away from the doctors and keep your financial status in perfect health. It can be quiet expensive to eat locally or get food from a local source, but it is always worth it to go the extra mile.

You can also raise your own chickens if you have the space. My mother raised the chickens we consumed. It was such a family treat! I always have a smile on my face each time I take a trip down to memory lane. Every Saturday, I was in charge of feeding them and collecting their eggs along with my siblings. My mother brought the farm to us and it was very educational and pleasurable spending our Saturdays with her. I was also in charge of attending the chickens and overlooking the crops in our small garden. Collecting ripe vegetables was a family affair every weekend then she taught us how to cut them and to consume them to taste the flavor in every bite we took.

It is legal in hundreds of cities in the United States to raise your own animals or birds, but always contact the mayor's office to know the *do's* and *don'ts*. If you do, make sure you keep your chickens within limit and take care of them regularly. If that sounds like too much work, there is a butcher waiting for you at a Whole Foods Market location or your local farmer.

Our food consumption should include the following:

1. Find a reliable, cost-effective and long-term local farmland. See how their meat is raised and study the farmer himself or herself. Invest in them and you will soon reap the benefits of eating healthy.
2. Do not only purchase your meat or produce locally, but also try to purchase your dairy products such as milk, jellies, peanut butter, beans, etc., from them as well.
3. Protect yourself from the industrial system. Most supermarkets are full of them. Shoppers from those supermarkets always think about what to eat now instead of focusing on how the meat is raised and where it comes from?
4. Help a family member, fellow neighbor or a friend eat healthy and refer them to your farmer(s). Teach them why it is important to eat food close to their homes and let them taste your food.
5. Last but not least, inform yourself and others around you about local consumerism and learn enough about it and pass it down to your offspring. They will be grateful you did just as I am towards my mother. By getting your children to taste your local farm's

meat, they will think twice before buying that *cardboard* tasting meat that is supplied in our restaurants, schools etc.

6. Reduce the amount of meat you consume each week to once a week or once a month. Your health will be grateful you did.

After adopting to follow these principles I have lost more weight and felt much healthier than I previously was. I cannot claim that you will get the same results, but I am sure you will feel healthy, lighter and enjoy more of the foods you consume. Nowadays, there are chefs who mainly use local ingredients and are willing to teach their customers about the benefits of local eating and how to cook them. You have to support the institutions that feed us in schools, the workplace, hospitals, etc., to use fresh, natural, wholesome foods. Here is what to do:

1. Find a farmer who fits your criteria and stick with him or her for the long haul. Listen to him or her when he or she is conversing and suggest your approaches.
2. Make field trips with your family to see how their food is made.
3. Commit to seasonal foods and cook your way around it. There are thousands of recipes online that you can use or purchase a cookbook from your local bookstore.
4. Teach yourself how to eat nutritionally and medicinally rich food to avoid the painful effects in the near future.

The government has decimated the growth of local and wholesome foods to nourish us. It's up to us to regain control of what goes in the foods we consume and ask the USDA to subsidize our local farmers to make our local food more affordable. This will liberate thousands of young farmers who want to farm for a living to free us from the systematic foods that we have long consumed. These young farmers have no choice but to step back because there are not enough investors to back them up in the healthy farming sectors. Many of the subsidies only go to those opting for cheap food, devaluing our farmers instead of uplifting them. By supporting the large-scale food distribution system, you are devaluing our small-scale farmers who have no choice but to step back. Less than 2% of Americans farm for a living, a frightening statistic. The average age of a farmer is 50 years old. If no one steps in to push the government to change its habit, who will farm for us in the next decade? We have to urge the government to rebuild the ancient infrastructure that we have long forgotten to heal us so we can live to meet our great grandchildren. Supporting naturally and locally grown food is simple. Here is how:

1. We can step in to donate to our local farmers ourselves to encourage them to farm. We can also use our connections (government officials) to support them.
2. We can organize fundraisers or create donation websites to support our local farmers.
3. We can help them write their business plans to attract investors.
4. We can listen, support, and coach them in their endeavors.
5. We can lend our lands for a small fee or donate them if possible.
6. We can help them campaign or lobby to push the government to subsidize them.
7. We can use our own capital and expertise to build infrastructures to help them.
8. We can invest in a local farmer in an exchange of seasonal crops delivered to our home.
9. We have to support them in a spirit of collaboration to help them get off their feet.
10. We can build institutions to help veteran farmers teach the youngsters how to farm.

If adopted, we can have a sustainable farmland in no time with thousands of options to choose from and at the same time discourage the industrialization system. Eating smartly does not have to be difficult. It is up to us to determine what our permanent fixture in healthy eating is. As long as life is still going on, we have to adapt to a healthy approach not just thinking about our pockets alone. My father always tells me: *When there is health, anything is possible.* As I keep on repeating throughout the book, you reap what you sow thus the more we adapt to a healthier life, the happier we will be. It is been a privilege to learn a little about our Western diet and healthy eating and share it with you. I have always been fond of learning new things. Those around me know how I can react whenever they are consuming an unhealthy food. What I show them is my shaved head and that is enough for them to throw their food in the garbage. The question you have to ask yourself is: *Do I want my food to be produced naturally or in a laboratory?* It is such an honor to learn and care a lot more about nutrition and share it with you on behalf of the fertility of our soils. The earth is a blessing and it is up to us to use it to heal and protect ourselves. Whenever you are cooking with food that is alive such as vegetables and fruits (pesticides and chemicals free), you are no longer in danger of collecting chemical nutrients or any other harmful effects. Health is never for sale, so why cheapen it with unhealthy habits? Commit to making the change today and reap the benefits of the soil. Local is for the betterment of our society, not the other way around. As a new food activist, I believe everyone have the right to food democracy. Local, organic, nontoxic, healthy are all the components that are needed in a food. That kind of food is the populist appeal and sooner or later, healthy eating will overcome the industrial revolution that you've long been suffering from. It's been a privilege to share this little knowledge with you. I hope you put it in a great use.

Acknowledgments

I will be curt offering my gratitude as I have it for thousands. First to my father Tchaisso, without whom I wouldn't have the knowledge today that I have acquired. He is my hero, my teacher, the wisest and the most successful entrepreneur I have ever known. Dad has always believed in me and never has his faith been shaken when it came to me. I would also like to thank my mother (my Queen), Beatrice, the *feeder* of our humble family. She is the greatest and most beautiful woman I have ever encountered. I am lucky enough to call her my mother. As kids, we have always pushed her meals aside because it was "meatless" as we called it but as tough as she is, we always had to do as "she says". We hated her for it but as the fully grown woman that I am today, I am grateful for her teachings about smart eating. I would like to extend my gratitude to my brothers Jules and Edik Although my brothers and I are as different as night and day, it is a privilege for me to refer to them as my family. They have always been my healthy competitors. To my dearest princess and sister, Sonie who not only filled my lonely heart, but always brought a smile on my face each time I hear her voice. She always pushed me to behave accordingly as she watched my steps carefully. She does not like me gushing over her but I cannot help myself. I am glad she has grown into such a lovely young woman.

I also extend my gratitude to my best friend and life coach, Tom, for his guidance and care in my desperate moments. He never shook on his words and always goes straight to the point. He is the greatest man I have ever met, although we sometimes face disparities, he surely knows how the calm my windy days. We laugh less, but his faith and support has never changed. His teaching routine has kept me going when my legs are still and when my lips refuse to be parted. For all those things and also for being my muse, I thank you. I would not have had the courage to write my first word if it was not for you, Tom. Your encouragements were always there to carry me through my two years of writing. I would also like to thank my best friends Xenobia and Khadija Derrouche for their love and support, which have never faded. Khadija, no matter where you are, you will always be known as the woman who saved my life. I will forever be thankful. To my editor Nicholas, the CEO of Twin Miracles Editorial, my words cannot express my gratitude. You have protected my work and worked on it as if it was your own, I am looking forward to working with you on my upcoming projects!

We oftentimes call our dearest people our friends, but I consider them my godsends. I believe they have been sent to guide, cheer and help me by the divine. I am profoundly grateful to those who helped in writing, editing and publishing his book. I shiver with awareness about those around me for their anticipation, their presence and their love in my life. There are more adventures in the future but I have an unshaken faith that my godsends will always be present.

List of Farmers Markets

California

There are thousands of farmers markets in California but I am just listing the ones I have visited. Feel free to look for other nearby markets. Enjoy!

Los Angeles and Nearby Counties

Mondays

- o Bellflower: Oak Street and Clark Avenue, 9:00 a.m. to 1:00 p.m. (562) 866-6609.
- o South Gate: South Gate Park, Tweedy Boulevard and Pinehurst Avenue, 9:00 a.m. to 1:00 p.m. (323) 774-0159.
- o West Hollywood: Plummer Park, north lot, 1200 N. Vista St. at Fountain Avenue, 9:00 a.m. to 2:00 p.m. (323) 848-6535.

Tuesdays

- o Culver City: Main Street between Venice and Culver Boulevards, 2:00 to 7:00 p.m. (310) 739-5028.
- o Highland Park: Marmion Way at Avenue fifty-seven (near Gold Line station), summer, 4:00 to 8:00 pm; winter, 3:00 to 7:00 p.m. www.oldla.org (323) 255-5030.
- o Manhattan Beach: Thirteen Street between Valley and Morningside Drives, noon to 5:00 p.m. Memorial Day through Labor Day. www.mbfarmersmarket.com. (310) 379-9901.

o   Norwalk: South side of Alondra Boulevard, west of Pioneer Boulevard, 9:00 a.m. to 1:00 p.m. (562) 921-2321.

o   Pasadena (Villa Park): 363 E. Villa St. at Garfield Avenue, 8:30 a.m. to 12:30 p.m. (626) 449-0179.

o   Torrance: Wilson Park on Crenshaw Boulevard, between Carson Street and Sepulveda Boulevard, 8:00 a.m. to 1:00 p.m. (310) 781-7520.

o   Brea: Birch Street and Walnut Avenue, 4:00 to 8:30 p.m. during daylight savings time, 4:00 to 8:00 p.m. the remainder of the year. (714) 329-6755.

o   Irvine: Historic Park at the Irvine Ranch, 13042 Old Myford Road, 9:00 a.m. to 1:00 p.m. (714) 573-0374.

o   Big Bear Lake: Big Bear Boulevard and Division Road, April through October, 8:30 a.m. to 1:00 p.m. (760) 247-3769.

Wednesdays

o   Gardena: 1670 W.162nd St., 9:00 a.m. to 1:00 p.m. (310) 217-9537.

o   Hollywood (Sears): 5601 Santa Monica Boulevard, noon to 5:30 p.m. (EBT) (323) 463-3171.

o   Huntington Park: Salt Lake City Park, Bissell Street and East Florence Avenue, 9:30 a.m. to 1:30 p.m. (866) 466-3834.

o   La Cienega (Kaiser): Kaiser West LA, 6041 Cadillac Ave., 9:00 a.m. to 1:30 p.m. (EBT) (562) 495-1764.

o   Lawndale: 147th Street and Hawthorne Boulevard at City Hall, 2:00 to 7:00 p.m. (310) 679-3306.

o   Los Angeles (Adams and Vermont): St. Agnes Church, West Adams Boulevard at Vermont Avenue, 2:00 to 6:00 p.m. (EBT) (323) 777-1755.

o   Los Angeles (downtown): 650 W. 5th St., 11:30 a.m. to 2:00 p.m. (EBT) www.ccfm.com. (818) 591-8161.

o   Northridge: Northridge Fashion Center, Tampa Avenue south of Plummer Street, April through October 24, 5:00 to 9:00 p.m. (805) 643-6458.

o   San Dimas: 245 E. Bonita Ave., 5:00 to 9:00 p.m., April 2 through September 24. (909) 581-4744.

o Santa Monica: Second Street and Arizona Avenue, 8:30 a.m. to 1:30 p.m. (EBT) www.smgov.net/farmers_market. (310) 458-8712.

o Westchester: Westchester Park at Lincoln Boulevard and La Tijera, 8:30 a.m. to 1:00 p.m. www.westchesterfarmersmarket.com. (310) 582-5850.

o Whittier: Greenleaf Avenue between Philadelphia and Hadley Streets. March 5 through Third week in October, 5:00 to 9:00 p.m. (562) 696-2662.

o Chino Hills: McCoy Equestrian Center, 14280 Peyton Drive, 4:00 to 8:30 p.m. April 2 through September 24. (909) 548-0868.

Thursdays

o Parking lot, Carson Street between Bonita Street and Avalon Boulevard, 9:00 a.m. to 1:00 p.m. (310) 847-3584.

o Century City: Constellation Boulevard and Avenue of the Stars, 11:30 a.m. to 3:00 p.m. www.ccfm.com. (818) 591-8161.

o El Segundo: Main Street between Holly and Pine Avenues, 3:00 to 7:00 p.m. (310) 615-2649.

o Glendale: 100 block of North Brand, between Wilson Avenue and Broadway Boulevard, 9:30 a.m. to 1:30 p.m. (818) 548-2005.

o Glendora: 140 S. Glendora Ave., 5:00 to 9:00 p.m. May 1 through August 28. (626) 593-9254.

o La Cienega: La Cienega Plaza, 1801 S. La Cienega Blvd., 3:00 to 7:00 p.m.; 3:00 to 7:30 p.m. during daylight savings time. (EBT) (562) 495-1764.

o La Verne: Old Town La Verne, D Street and Bonita Avenue, April 3 through August 28. 5:00 to 9:00 p.m. (626) 357-7442.

o Long Beach (Uptown): Atlantic Ave and E 45th Way (Bixby Knolls area) 3:00 to 6:30 p.m. (EBT) (866) 466-3834.

o Los Angeles (Chinatown): 727 N. Hill St., 2:00 to 6:00 p.m. www.chinatownla.com. (213) 680-0243.

o Redondo Beach: Adjacent to Veterans Park, 309 Esplanade at the pier, 8:00 a.m. to 1:00 p.m. (310) 372-1171, ext. 2252.

o Newhall: Market between Walnut and Main, 3:00 to 7:00 p.m. (661) 255-4347.

o Westwood: Sepulveda Boulevard at Constitution Avenue (just north of Wilshire), noon to 6:00 p.m. (until sunset in winter) (310) 861-8188.

o Wilmington: Avalon Boulevard and L Street, 9:00 a.m. to 1:00 p.m. (310) 834-8586.

o Anaheim: Center Street Promenade at Lemon Street, 9:00 a.m. to 1:30 p.m. (EBT) (714) 956-3586.

o Costa Mesa: Orange County Fairgrounds, 88 Fair Drive, 9:00 a.m. to 1:00 p.m. (714) 573-0374.

o Fullerton: Wilshire Avenue between Harbor Boulevard and Pomona Avenue, 4:00 to 8:30 p.m. April through November. (714) 738-6545.

o Orange: 143 S. Lemon St., American Legion Hall parking lot, 2:00 to 6:00 p.m. (951) 532-2822.

o Redlands: East State Street between Orange and Ninth Streets, 6:00 to 9:00 p.m.; summer hours, May 31 to September 4: 6:00 to 9:30 p.m. (909) 798-7629.

o Upland: Ninth Street and Second Avenue, April to late October, 5:00 to 9:00 p.m. (714) 345-3087.

o Victorville (High Desert): Victor Valley Community College Upper Campus, 8:00 a.m. to noon. (760) 247-3769.

o Oxnard: Plaza Park, corner of Fifth and C Streets, 9:00 a.m. to 1:00 p.m. (805) 483-7960.

o Thousand Oaks: McCloud Avenue and Hillcrest Drive, 403 W. Hillcrest Dr., on the rooftop of Conejo Recreation and Park District building, 2:00 to 6:30 p.m. www.vccfarmersmarkets.com. (805) 529-6266.

Fridays

o Covina: Civic Center Park, Citrus Avenue and School Street, 5:00 to 9:00 p.m. April through December. www.covinafarmersmarket. com. (310) 621-0336.

o Echo Park: Parking lot no. 663 on Logan Street south of Sunset Boulevard, 3:00 to 7:00 p.m. (EBT) (323) 463-3171.

o Long Beach (downtown): CityPlace, on the Promenade between Fourth and Fifth Streets, 10:00 a.m. to 4:00 p.m. (EBT). (866) 466-3834.

o Los Angeles (downtown): 333 S. Hope St., 11:00 a.m. to 2:00 p.m. (818) 591-8161.

o Los Angeles (Eagle Rock): Merton and Caspar Avenues, 5:00 to 9:00 p.m.

o Monrovia: East Olive and South Myrtle Avenues, 5:00 to 9:00 p.m. January 4 through December 19. (626) 357-7442.

o San Pedro: Old Town, Mesa and sixth streets, 9:00 a.m. to 2:00 p.m. (310) 832-7272.

o Simi Valley: Simi Valley Town Center Mall, 1555 Simi Town Center Way, March through November, 3:00 to 8:00 p.m. (805) 643-6458.

o Venice: Venice Way and Venice Boulevard, 7:00 to 11:00 a.m. www.venicefarmersmarket.com. (310) 399-6690.

o Whittier: Bailey Street between Greenleaf and Comstock Avenues, 8:00 a.m. to 1:00 p.m. (EBT) (562) 696-2662.

Saturdays

o Burbank: Orange Grove Avenue and Third Street, behind City Hall, 8:00 a.m. to 12:30 p.m. (EBT) (626) 308-0457.

o Calabasas (Old Town): 23504 Calabasas Road, at Mulholland Drive, 8:00 a.m. to 1:00 p.m. www.ccfm.com. (818) 591-8161.

o Cerritos: Park Plaza and Towne Center Drives, near the Performing Arts Center, 8:00 a.m. to noon. (EBT) (866) 466-3834.

o Gardena: Hollypark United Methodist Church parking lot, 13,000 S. Van Ness Ave., 6:30 a.m. to 12:30 p.m. (EBT) (323) 777-1755.

o La Cañada Flintridge: 1346 Foothill Blvd., across from Memorial Park, 9:00 a.m. to 1:00 p.m. www.ccfm.com. (818) 591-8161.

o Leimert: Degnan Boulevard and Forty Third Street, 10:00 a.m. to 3:00 p.m. (EBT) (323) 463-3171.

o Los Angeles (Harambee): 5730 Crenshaw Blvd., north of Slauson Avenue, 10:00 a.m. to 4:00 p.m. (323) 292-5550; (323) 292-5558.

o Pasadena (Victory Park): North Sierra Madre Boulevard and Paloma Street, 8:30 a.m. to 12:30 p.m. (EBT) (626) 449-0179.

o Pomona Valley: Pearl Street and Garey Avenue, 7:30 to 11:30 a.m. (EBT) (310) 621-0336.

o Santa Monica (Pico): Virginia Avenue Park, corner of Pico and Cloverfield Boulevards, 8:00 a.m. to 1:00 p.m. (EBT) (310) 458-8712.

o Santa Monica (Saturday, organic): Third Street at Arizona Avenue, 8:30 a.m. to 1:00 p.m. (EBT) www.smgov.net/farmers_market. (310) 458-8712.

o Silver Lake: 3700 Sunset Blvd., 8:00 a.m. to 1:00 p.m. (323) 661-7771.

o Torrance: Wilson Park, 2200 Crenshaw Blvd., 8:00 a.m. to 1:00 p.m. (310) 328-2809.

o Walnut: Southlands Christian School campus, 1920 S. Brea Canyon Cutoff Road., 8:00 a.m. to 1:00 p.m. (909) 860-1904.

o Westchester: Promenade at Howard Hughes Center, 6081 Center Dr. 8:30 a.m. to 1:00 p.m. www.westchesterfarmersmarket.com. (310) 582-5850.

o Corona Del Mar: Marguerite Avenue and Pacific Coast Highway, 9:00 a.m. to 1:00 p.m. (949) 361-0735.

o Dana Point: Hennessey's La Plaza, Pacific Coast Highway and Golden Lantern, 9:00 a.m. to 1:00 p.m. (909) 229-3329.

o Irvine: University Center across from UCI, 8:00 a.m. to noon. (714) 573-0374.

o Ladera Ranch: Town Green Park, 28801 Sienna Parkway, 9:00 a.m. to 1:00 p.m.

Sundays

o Alhambra: Monterey and East Bay State Streets, 8:30 a.m. to 1:00 p.m. (EBT) (626) 570-5081.

o Atwater: 3250 Glendale Blvd., 10:00 a.m. to 2:00 p.m. (EBT) (323) 463-3171.

o Beverly Hills: 9300 block of Civic Center Drive, 9:00 a.m. to 1:00 p.m. (310) 285-6830.

o   Brentwood: 741 Gretna Green Way, at San Vicente Boulevard, 9:00 a.m. to 2:30 p.m. www.ccfm.com. (818) 591-8161.

o   Claremont: Second Street and Indian Hill Boulevard, 8:00 a.m. to 1:00 p.m. (714) 345-3087.

o   Encino: 17400 Victory Blvd., 8:00 a.m. to 1:00 p.m. (818) 708-6611. Hollywood: Ivar Avenue between Sunset and Hollywood Boulevards, 8:00 a.m. to 1:00 p.m. (EBT) (323) 463-3171.

o   Long Beach (Southeast): Parking lot of the Alamitos Bay Marina, East Marina Drive, south of East Second Street, west of Pacific Coast Highway, 9:00 a.m. to 2:00 p.m. (EBT) (866) 466-3834.

o   Los Angeles (Larchmont Village): 209 Larchmont Blvd., between First Street and Beverly Boulevard, 10:00 a.m. to 2:00 p.m. (818) 591-8161.

o   Los Angeles (Melrose Place): Melrose Place and Melrose Avenue, 10:00 a.m. to 2:00 p.m. (818) 591-8161.

o   Mar Vista: Venice Boulevard and Grand View Boulevard, Los Angeles, 9:00 a.m. to 2:00 p.m. (310) 861-4444.

o   Montrose (Harvest Market): 2200 block of Honolulu Avenue, 9:00 a.m. to 2:00 p.m. (818) 249-2499.

o   Santa Clarita: College of the Canyons, stadium parking lot 8, Valencia and Rockwell Canyon Boulevards, 8:30 a.m. to noon. (805) 529-6266.

o   Santa Monica: 2640 Main St. at Ocean Park Boulevard, 9:30 a.m. to 1:00 p.m. (EBT) (310) 458-8712.

o   Studio City: Ventura Place, between Ventura and Laurel Canyon Boulevards, 8:00 a.m. to 1:00 p.m. (818) 655-7744.

o   West Los Angeles: 11360 Santa Monica Blvd., at Purdue Avenue, behind the public library, 9:00 a.m. to 2:00 p.m. (310) 281-7855.

o   Westwood Village: Broxton Avenue between Weyburn and Kinross Avenues, 10:00 a.m. to 3:00 p.m. (310) 739-5028.

o   San Clemente Village: Avenida Del Mar and Ola Vista, 9:00 a.m. to 1:00 p.m. (949) 361-0735.

o   Fullerton: Independence Park, 801 W. Valencia Ave. (next to DMV), 8:00 a.m. to 1:30 p.m. (714) 871-5304.

o   San Juan Capistrano: El Camino Real and Yorba Lane, 3:00 to 7:00 p.m. (858) 272-7054.

- o Santa Ana: Fiesta Marketplace parking lot, North Bush and East Third Streets, 3:00 to 7:00 p.m. www.grainproject.org. (714) 542-9392.
- o Tustin: El Camino Real and Third Street, 9:00 a.m. to 1:00 p.m. (714) 573-0374.
- o Temecula (Promenade): Promenade Mall, 4820 Winchester Rd at Inez Road, 9:00 a.m. to 1:00 p.m. (760) 728-7343.
- o Chino: Chino City Hall, 13220 Central Ave., June through August 5:00 to 8:30 p.m. www.chinofarmersmarket.com. (310) 621-0336.
- o Ventura (midtown): Pacific View Mall, west lot, north of Sears, 9:00 a.m. to 1:00 p.m. www.vccfarmersmarkets.com. (805) 529-6266.
- o Huntington Beach: Pier Plaza, Main Street and Pacific Coast Highway, 1:00 to 5:00 p.m. (714) 573-0374.
- o Laguna Hills: Laguna Hills Mall parking lot, the 5 Freeway and El Toro Road, 9:00 a.m. to 1:00 p.m. (714) 573-0374.

Pennsylvania

Pennsylvania has many farmers markets, large and small, offering a selection of fresh produce and numerous other products. Most farmers markets are open seasonally, and some year-round. You can also visit your local Produce Junction Market. They are wholesalers and sell their goods at the fraction of the cost of grocery stores. They mostly carry fruits and vegetables. Visit their website: www.producejuction.com to find the nearest. For fresh meat, visit Vivero Albaraka Farm. They are located on: 1425 West Lycoming Street, Philadelphia, PA (215) 226-6666 or (215) 226-2601 or www.albarakafarm.com. With this farm, you have the option to choose your livestock or poultry before the slaughter. They have all kind of animals or birds you might be seeking. They are open seven days a week from 8:00 a.m. to 7:00 p.m. Delivery options are also available.

For Philadelphia County: 2241 Bryn Mawr Ave, Philadelphia, PA 19131 (215) 477-5007

Philadelphia County

o Fair Food Farm Stand (12th and Arch in Center City), Philadelphia at the Reading Terminal Market on the 12th Street. Opens Monday-Saturday, 8:00 a.m.-6:00 p.m. & Sunday 9:00 a.m.-5:00 p.m. (215) 627-2029. Year Round!

o Reading Terminal Market (Fifty-First North Twelfth Street) opens Monday to Saturday, 8:00 a.m.-6:00 p.m. Contact Information: www.readingterminalmarket.org (215) 922-2317

o Broad and South farmers market opens (May-October) Broad & South Street, 2:00-7:00 pm on Wednesdays (215) 575-0444

o Fairmount Market (Twenty-Second Street and Fairmount Avenue) opens May 5 through November 17, 3:00 to 7:00 p.m. on Thursdays.

o Germantown Market (Germantown Avenue and Walnut Lane) opens May to November 20, 2:00 to 6:00 p.m. on Fridays.

o Phoenixville Market (Under the Gay Street Bridge, accessible via Taylor Alley) opens May 7 through November 19, 9:00 a.m.

to 1:00 p.m. on Saturdays; in winter, 10:00 to 11:30 a.m. two Saturday per month.

o Doylestown Market (Hamilton and West State Streets) opens April 16 to November 19, 7:00 a.m. to noon on Saturdays.

o Rittenhouse Market (Eighteenth and Walnut Streets) opens December to April, 10:00 a.m. to 2:00 p.m. on Saturdays; May to November, 10 a.m. to 1:00 p.m. on Tuesdays and 9:30 a.m. to 3:00 p.m. on Saturdays.

o University Square Market (Thirty-Six and Walnut Streets) opens May through Thanksgiving (November), 10:00 a.m. to 3:00 p.m. on Wednesdays.

o Clark Park Market (Forty-Third Street and Baltimore Avenue) opens year-round, 10:00 a.m. to 2:00 p.m. on Saturdays, and June 2 to November 17th, 3:00 to 7:00 p.m. on Thursdays.

o Collingswood Market (along Atlantic Avenue between Collings and Irvin Avenues) Open May 7 to November 19, 8:00 a.m. to noon on Saturdays.

o Bryn Mawr Market (Lancaster and Morris Avenues). Open April 23 through October, 9:00 a.m. to 1:00 p.m. on Saturdays; November through April, every fourth Saturday.

o South & Passyunk Market (South Street and Passyunk Avenue, just east of Fifth Street).Open Mid-May to November 22nd, 2:30 to 7 p.m. on Tuesdays

o West Chester Growers Markets, church and Chestnut Streets, May through November, 9:00a.m. 1:00p.m on Saturdays.

Lancaster County

o Bird-in-Hands farmers markets (Bird-in-Hand, PA). (717) 393-9674

o Cherry Hill Orchards, Inc. (Lancaster PA). (717) 872-9311

o Fisher's Bakery & Roadside Stand (Gordonville, PA). (7171) 768-3541

o Green Dragon farmers market & Auction (Ephrata, PA). (717) 738-1117 o   Kauffman's Fruits Farm and Market (Bird-in-Hand, PA). (717) 768-7112

o   Lancaster Central Market (Lancaster PA). (717) 735-6890

o   Oasis at Bird-in-Hand (Ronks, PA). (717) 288-2154

o   Stoudt's Wonderful Good Market. (Adamstown PA). (717) 484-4386

o   Village Farm Market (Ephrata, PA). (717) 733-5340

Farms Stands in Pennsylvania

o   The farm stands of the Greater Pittsburgh Community Food Bank open June 10 and run through November 12. The Farm Stand Project provides affordable produce to low-income neighborhoods that have limited access to grocery stores. Farm-stand specialist Vicki Lish says they're aiming to add more local produce this year.

o   They added one stand-Charles Street on the North Side, sponsored by the Pittsburgh Project-and closed two: Lincoln-Larimer and East Hills.

All stands, which are sponsored by community groups and run by local residents, accept cash, WIC, senior farmers market Nutrition Program vouchers, and food stamps. Most have a grand opening the week of July 6.

Wednesday Farm Stands

o   Mon Yough Community Services, 500 Market St., McKeesport (Market Street at Fifth Avenue), 9:30 a.m. to 1:30 p.m.

o   Seton Brookline, 1900 Pioneer Ave., Brookline (Elizabeth Seton Center lot), 11:00 a.m. to 6:00 p.m.

o   Turtle Creek Valley, 519 Penn Ave., Turtle Creek (in front of the WVHSC building), noon to 3:00 p.m.

o   Millvale, 400 Grant Ave. (in the rear lot), 3:00 to 6:30 p.m.

Thursday Farm Stands

o   Homewood-Brushton YMCA, 7140 Bennett St., Homewood, 12:30 to 6:30 p.m.

- o Hill House, 1835 Centre Ave., Hill District (next to main entrance), 10:00 a.m. to 1:00 p.m.
- o Addison Terrace, 2136 Elmore Square (across from Addison Community Center), 11:00 a.m. to 3:00 p.m.
- o Hazelwood YMCA, 4915 Second Ave. (Dairy Mart lot), 11:30 a.m. to 2:30 p.m.
- o Clairton, 530 Miller Ave. (Lifespan Senior Center), 10:30 a.m. to 1:30 p.m.
- o Lawrenceville, 286 Main St. (Stephen Foster Center), 11:30 a.m. to 2:30 p.m.
- o Charles Street, 2801 N. Charles St., North Side (at Fowler Park), 2:00 to 6:00 p.m.

For More Farm Stand Markets, Please call: (412) 460-3663

New Jersey

New Jersey has many farmers' markets, large and small, offering a selection of fresh produce and numerous other products. Most farmers' markets are open seasonally, and some year-round. For more information on farmers' markets in New Jersey, visit: www.localharvest.org

Washington Township farmers' market

Operation Date and Time: Sundays, mid-June to September (Knights of Columbus, 79 Pascack Road).

Reasons to go: This farmers' market includes Jersey fresh fruits and vegetables, breads, pies, pastries, pasta, sauces, cheeses, pickles, pickled vegetables, fudge, baklava, plants, flowers, and more.

Fort Lee farmers market

Operation Time and Date: Sundays, June to November and it is located on the Community Center off Anderson Avenue

Reasons to go: Fresh fruits and vegetables, artisan breads and cheeses, pickles, plants, pies and more.

Paramus farmers market

Operation Time and Date: Late June through September. Located on the Petruska Memorial Park's North Parking Lot

Reasons to go: Jersey fresh fruits and vegetables, bakery and breads, homemade pasta and sauces, handmade mozzarella, Italian sausages, pickles and olives, jellies and James, kielbasa, and bratwurst, and a dog bakery.

Emerson farmers market

Operation Time and Date: Sundays, late June to November. Borough of Emerson 1 Municipal Place Emerson, NJ 07630 (201) 297-4156

Reasons to go: The Orchards of Conklin from Rockland County is here and aside from their freshly grown fruit, they bring their freshly baked pies and donuts. There are additional farm stands with a large selection of fresh fruits and vegetables, including white carrots, which are sweeter than the orange ones, and freshly picked mushrooms. There are pickles, freshly made mozzarella, and artisan breads.

Ramsey farmers market

Operation hours and Dates: Sundays, early-June to November (Ramsey Train Station, Erie Plaza off Main Street).

Reasons to go: Fresh fish from Hampton Bays, organic fruits and vegetables, Orchards of Conklin, fresh cut flowers, Dr. Pickles, organic teas and coffees, homespun chili, Ventimiglia Vineyards, quiches, gluten-free bakery items, goat milk cheeses, artisan breads, jams, fresh pies, fresh pastas, honey and so much more!

Ridgewood farmers market

Operation Time and Dates: Sundays, late June to November (Ridgewood Train Station).

Reasons to go: There's a fresh honey stand for honey lovers, homemade jams, fresh breads and pies, pickles and of course, a huge selection of fresh fruits and vegetables as well as a large selection of fresh herbs.

Tenafly farmers market

Operation Time and Date: Sundays, now through October (parking lot at the corner of Tenafly Road and Washington Street).

Why Go: Large selection of organic fruits, vegetables and an organic bread stand. In addition to the organic stands, there are two large vegetable stands, a plant/flower stand, freshly made goat's milk cheeses, a featured artist and a kids' art table.

Hasbrouck Heights farmers market

Operation Time and Date: Tuesdays, mid-June through September. It is located on the Corner of Boulevard and Central Avenue

Reasons to go: There are two farm stands offering fruits and vegetables, an organic bakery, pickles, mozzarella, breads, fresh ravioli and a stand that sells organic handmade soap.

Haworth farmers market

Operation Time and Dates: Daily Tuesdays, early-June to November (Terrace Street parking lot)

Reasons to go: Farm-fresh fruits, vegetables, pickles, olives, breads, cheeses and more.

Rutherford-Farmers' Market

Operation Time and Dates: Wednesdays and Saturdays, June through October (Williams Plaza).

Reasons to go: The Wednesday market features Jersey fresh produce from two New Jersey farms, Amish-baked goods, pickles, frozen seafood and pasta, dried fruits and nuts, and an assortment of other products. The Saturday market only features New Jersey fresh farm produce.

River Vale Farmers' Market

Operation Time and Dates: Daily Thursdays late-June through October (River Vale Town Hall Complex, 406 Rivervale Road, in the parking lot next to the tennis courts).

Reasons to go: It has a lot of vendors, including two fresh fruit and vegetable stands, one of which is Stokes Farm from Old Tappan; a handmade wine stand—with tastings! (If you like wine, try theirs!); a stand that offers handmade sodas and coffees; a stand with fresh handmade pasta sauces and pizzas; a fresh Italian ice stand; a pickle stand; an Amish stand with all the amazing homemade pies, pastries, and jams, and a fresh mozzarella and bread stand.

Teaneck farmers market

Operation Time and Dates: Thursdays, mid-June through October, Municipal parking lot off Cedar Lane, Garrison Avenue and Beverly Road, in back of the Wells Fargo Bank (across from Bischoff's).

Reasons to go: There are two farm stands, but one of them is Amish, and you have never seen such enormous vegetables or a stand so perfectly arranged with endless offerings. And don't forget to take home some Amish baked goods like whoopee pies, snicker-doodles, or jams. There's also a mozzarella and bread stand and a pickle stand.

Englewood farmers market

Operation Time and Dates: Fridays, mid-June through October and it is located on Depot Square off North Van Brunt Street.

Reasons to go: Stands with a wide variety of fruits and vegetables, an Amish stand with homemade baked goods, a mozzarella and bread stand, and pickles.

Hawthorne farmers market

Operation Time and Dates: Sundays, late June through October. Grand Avenue between Jefferson Place and McKinley Avenue (behind the library)

Reasons to go: Fresh fruits and vegetables, baked goods, meats, cheeses and nuts.

Ringwood Farmers' Market

Operation Time and Dates: Saturdays, late May through October. Ringwood Park & Ride, Cannici Drive at Skyline Drive.

Reasons to go: Locally grown fruits and vegetables, eggs, honey, meats, Italian specialties, soup, locally roasted coffee, olives, artisan breads, cider, donuts, pulled pork and barbecue ribs, hummus, and kielbasa.

West Milford farmers market

Operation Time and Dates: Wednesdays, mid-June through October (Wells Fargo Bank Parking Lot, 1 Marshall Hill Road).

Reasons to go: Fruits, vegetables, baked goods, pickles, herbs and vegetables, plants, meats, eggs, jams and jellies, and Italian foods.

Hoboken Farmers' Market

Operation Time and Dates: Tuesdays, late June to November (Washington Street between Newark St. and Observer Highway).

Reasons to go: Variety of fruits and vegetables, baked goods, and pickles.

Hoboken Uptown Farmers' Market

Operation Time and Dates: Thursdays, early June through October (Hudson Street between Thirteenth and Fourteenth Streets).

Reasons to go: Variety of fruits and vegetables, baked goods, and pickles.

New York

New York City has many farmers' markets, large and small, offering a selection of fresh produce products. Most farmers' markets are open seasonally, and some year-round. Here is a list of the farmers markets I have visited in New York City.

77th Street Greenmarket

Operation hours and Dates: Sundays, 8:00 a.m. to 4:00 p.m. Columbus Avenue between 77th and 79th Streets.

Tribeca Greenmarket

Operation hours and Dates: Saturdays. Greenwich Street between Chambers and Duane

Reasons to go: Fresh fish and sheep's milk cheese.

Tucker Square Greenmarket

Operation dates and Time: Thursdays and Saturdays, 8:00 a.m. to 5:00 p.m. Columbus Avenue at 66th Street. Reasons to go: Enjoy this farmers market with cooking demonstrations and recipe exchanges

Tompkins Square Greenmarket

Sundays, 8:00 a.m. to 6:00 p.m. Avenue A and East Seventh Street

Reasons to go: Traditional farmers market at the Dag Hammarskjold Plaza.

Columbia Greenmarket

Operation Dates and Time: Thursdays and Sundays, 8:00 am to 5:00 pm Broadway between 114th and 115th Streets. Reasons to go: Shop with the students from Columbia University and staff of St. Luke's Hospital.

Bowling-Green Greenmarket

Tuesdays and Thursdays, 8:00 a.m. to 5:00 p.m. Broadway at Battery Place

Reasons to go: Purchase fresh fruit, quiches, and spring plants at this Lower Manhattan historic Bowling Green plaza.

Staten Island Ferry Whitehall Terminal Greenmarket

Operation Dates and Time: Tuesdays and Fridays, 8:00 a.m. to 7:00 p.m. 4 South Street, inside the ferry terminal building, Manhattan

Reasons to go: It is New York's first indoor greenmarket. At times, it includes activities and cooking demonstrations.

Notes and Abbreviations

Notes

Cals = calories

Fat = fat (fat level is valued in gram (g)).

Sat Fat = saturated fat (saturated fat level is valued in gram (g)).

Sugar = Sugar (sugar level is valued in gram (g)).

Sod = Sodium (sodium level is valued in milligram (mg)).

Chol = Cholesterol (cholesterol level is valued in gram (g)).

Carbs = Carbohydrate (carbohydrates level is valued in gram (g)).

Calci = calcium (calcium level is valued in milligram (mg)).

Fiber = fiber (fiber level is valued in gram (g)).

Prot = Protein (protein level is valued in gram (g)).

Potas = Potassium (Potassium level is valued in milligram (mg)).

Vit C = Vitamin C (Vitamin C level is valued in milligram (mg)).

"_____" (Dash) Indicates data no available.

0 (zero)= indicates that there is no nutrient in that food.

"< 1g" = less than 1 g of nutrient in that food.

Some figures are rounded values and may not be the same as label information from food manufacturers.

Abbreviations

Fl. = fluid

G= gram

Lb. = pounds

Pkg. = package

Serv. = serving

Tsp.= teaspoon

Oz. = ounce

Med = medium

Lg. = large

In = inch

Pt. = pint